To Allyson and Celina,
for the magic you bring into this world

DISCLAIMER

The content of this book is provided for general informational purposes only. The information is not intended or implied to be a substitute for medical advice, diagnosis, or treatment. It should not replace consultation with your physician or other qualified healthcare provider familiar with your individual health and medical needs.

Health and medical knowledge changes constantly. The information in this book should not be considered current, complete, or exhaustive. The content is not intended to establish any standard of care.

Never delay seeking professional medical advice or disregard it because of something you have read in this book. If you think you may have a medical emergency, call your doctor or 911 immediately.

The information presented herein represents the views of the author as of the date of publication. This book is presented for informational purposes only. Due to the rate at which conditions change, the author reserves the right to alter and update his opinions based on new conditions. While every attempt has been made to verify the information in this book, neither the author nor his affiliates/partners assume any responsibility for errors, inaccuracies, or omissions.

DAD LIVED TO 101 AND YOU CAN TOO

101 THINGS TO KNOW FOR HEALTH AND LONGEVITY

BILL TSU, MD

LIONCREST
PUBLISHING

DAD LIVED TO 101 AND YOU CAN TOO
101 *Things to Know for Health and Longevity*

ISBN   HARDCOVER: 978-1-5445-2865-6
       PAPERBACK: 978-1-5445-2866-3
       EBOOK: 978-1-5445-2867-0

CONTENTS

INTRODUCTION

On his hundredth birthday, my dad, Eddie, walked backward across his bedroom. Now, it wasn't as smooth as Michael Jackson's moonwalk, but it was still a wonderful sight to behold. Walking backward was one of the activities that kept Eddie fit as he aged. It's been practiced in Asia for centuries to promote the health of mind and body.

Even as a centenarian, my dad could recall both yesterday's dinner menu and stories of his children's antics from decades ago. Those who knew him would say that he retained his memory and wits because he was always reading and learning. It wasn't that simple, though. He took many other measures to keep his brain functioning well.

As a doctor, I watched with amazement at how well Eddie aged over the years. I was aware that this was partly because of his genes, but I also recognized that his longevity was primarily a result of how he lived his life. Over the course of this book, I will share with you Eddie's story so that you, too, can benefit from his healthy ways.

Whether you are young or old, already committed to maintaining your health or just starting out, this book is for you. It is never too late, or too early, to start thinking about longevity for yourself or your loved ones.

In Part 1 of this book, I will introduce the four pillars of a healthy lifestyle:

- eating for longevity
- staying physically active
- managing stress well
- avoiding unhealthy habits

A healthy lifestyle can delay or stop the onset of many illnesses and impairments of old age. It extends your life span, as well as your health span, which is the number of healthy years you live before a serious medical condition or the disabilities of aging affect your well-being. Eddie always said he was lucky to make it to 101, not only because of the number of years that he was alive, but because of the many healthy years that he had lived.

Eating for longevity is about more than just having a healthy diet. It's also about a way of eating that maintains a normal body weight. Eddie ate many nutritious foods, but along with these, he consumed plenty of white rice, a carbohydrate. Carbohydrates are blamed for much of the obesity problem and its associated medical conditions, but rice didn't hurt Eddie's waistline or his health. Learn why.

Staying physically active is one of the most important things you can do to live a long life. Doctors say that it's the best medicine there is. You can get enough physical activity without ever exercising—Eddie never exercised. Find out what activities helped to keep him healthy and fit.

Managing stress well is a common trait found in centenarians. For Eddie, the key was his perspective on life's events—the good and the unavoidable bad times. Three seemingly pessimistic expectations molded this perspective and were the basis for his happiness and low-stress existence.

Avoiding unhealthy habits can greatly affect your life span. Eddie had one, and he was lucky enough to live to an old age despite it. But many aren't so lucky. Smoking and excessive drinking are the two most common dangerous habits. I'm sure you are well aware that these behaviors are not good for you, but they deserve space in any book on longevity, because quitting either of them may be the best thing you can do to improve your chances of living a longer life. I've cared for thousands of smokers and drinkers in the operating room, so I've seen the damage firsthand. Hopefully, what I say will be one more reason to convince someone to break these addictions.

In Part 2 of this book, I will cover non-lifestyle practices and interventions that were essential for Eddie's longevity. Without them, I am sure he would not have lived to be a centenarian. These things to know are derived from my decades of experience working in hospitals and caring for my dad. They include the following:

- applying simple health concepts for detecting and preventing diseases
- taking advantage of physiological monitoring devices and techniques
- utilizing hospital-based measures to stay healthy
- understanding the aging process and its health implications

Applying simple health concepts can help you detect illnesses early and even prevent diseases. Among other things, applying these concepts involves acting on symptoms, keeping up with preventive care, and knowing how to make better healthcare decisions. Even as a physician, I once made the costly mistake of missing the significance of some innocent-appearing symptoms that Eddie developed when he was in his nineties. Instead of doing a medical workup, I blamed what he was experiencing on his advancing age. Don't make the same mistake—find out how to look at symptoms and catch problems earlier.

Taking advantage of physiologic monitoring devices and techniques is a smart health move. Something as simple as feeling a pulse can save a life or prevent a stroke. I have twice detected dangerous irregular heart rhythms in family members by using this simple maneuver. You can do it too. Learn this and the importance and nuances of employing other monitoring tools, such as a blood pressure machine and a pulse oximeter.

Utilizing hospital-based measures can prevent you from catching and spreading diseases. Discover how medically trained personnel practice these measures. They're helpful to know, not just in the time of COVID-19. They protected Eddie from the flu and other infections in his later years, when such illnesses could have been life-threatening.

In the final decade of Eddie's life, he and my mom moved into my home. This experience taught me firsthand about the day-to-day health concerns that many seniors face. It is important to be aware of age-related drug reactions, frailty from the loss of muscle mass, and even the problem of falling. Additionally, Eddie had clearly outlined his end-of-life wishes, and this knowledge guided me in caring for him in his final days.

It's a detailed journey, but also a valuable one. If you're looking for a concise and practical self-help book that can increase your chances of becoming a centenarian, then this book is it. Each chapter ends with a list of things to know to help you organize and remember the essential points.

Realize that in today's world, you have more control than ever over your health and longevity. It starts with believing in yourself and having the knowledge and will to do what is most beneficial for your well-being—not just for today, but for all the years ahead. So let's begin to live a healthier and longer life and help our loved ones do the same.

PART 1

LIVING A
HEALTHY LIFE

CHAPTER 1

HEALTHY EATING
WITH AN
UNREMARKABLE DIET

I walked briskly down the cookie aisle of the local super-market. I knew exactly where to go—toward the back of the store, right side, top shelf. Social Tea, Eddie's favorite cookie, had occupied this very location for years. I picked up a couple of boxes and placed them in my shopping cart, which held only soda cans, dark chocolate treats, and a big bag of potato chips—it was my monthly shopping trip for my dad's snacks.

EDDIE'S FOOD CHOICES

"What did your father eat?"

That's usually the first question I'm asked when someone learns that Eddie lived to be a centenarian. It's a good question, because what he ate did affect his health.

I wish I could tell you that he consumed a bowl of seaweed with each meal and drank five cups of ginseng tea every day, along with a few slices of ginger before bedtime. That if you do the same, you too will live a long and healthy life. The reality is that he did none of these things. In fact, his diet was quite simple. He ate traditional Chinese food for much of his life—his lunches and dinners usually consisted of white rice, a vegetable, and some tofu, fish, or chicken. But he also consumed a variety of American dishes after arriving in this country at the age of twenty-seven.

In my youth, my dad and the family treated hamburgers, pizza, and steak as food for special occasions. "Today we are having McDonald's to celebrate," Eddie said to me on several of my childhood birthdays. He enjoyed these meals as much as his children did, as it was a delightful break from his usual cuisine. Over time, he ate more Western food, and eventually it became a once- or twice-weekly event.

In between his meals, my father loved to snack. Cookies, chips, and chocolates were his prized choices, along with soda to drink. After he moved into my home when he was ninety-two, I took on the responsibility of shopping for these treats. At the beginning of each month, I would go to the local supermarket to buy his goodies—hence my knowledge of the exact location of the Social Tea cookies.

Until the day he passed, Eddie snacked daily. Yet, despite the snacking, he remained healthy and stayed lean and fit. How was this possible?

EAT BALANCED MEALS TO MEET YOUR BODY'S NEEDS

I have no doubt that what Eddie put on his plate contributed to him reaching his centenarian years. The fact that he stayed in good health and had the strength and stamina to be active throughout his life was evidence that the food he consumed provided enough of the various nutrients—protein, carbohydrates, fats, vitamins, and minerals—to meet his body's needs. He achieved this not by eating any miracle food products, but by simply following the basic dietary recommendation of eating balanced meals with a variety of nutritious items from the major food groups.

For his grains, this centenarian ate plenty of plain white rice, almost always with his lunches and dinners. Rice is a carbohydrate, a macronutrient that has been unfairly stigmatized. Carbs have been faulted for weight problems and their related health issues in this country. But carbs didn't harm Eddie, and the same is true for the Japanese population. They, too, eat plenty of rice and other carbs; in fact, percentage-wise, they dine on as much or more carbohydrates than Americans. Yet their obesity rate is one-tenth of ours, and they possess one of the longest life expectancies in the world. Clearly, carbohydrates are not always bad for you.

If rice wasn't served, Eddie ate Chinese noodles, and as he Westernized his food choices, he added breads and potatoes to the selection of carbohydrates he ate. Eating enough vegetables, which is a problem for many, was never a problem for my father. Since he grew up in Asia, where people ate lots of leafy green vegetables (mainly because they were plentiful and cheap), this nutrient-packed food group was always a large part of his meals. His number one choice was bok choy, but spinach, broccoli, and green beans became staples as his diet evolved. Along with the many vegetables that Eddie dined on, he also ate lots of fruits. He treated them as dessert and often finished off dinner with a plate of sliced apples or pears or his favorite, a bunch of grapes.

Although much of his protein came from plants, like tofu, edamame beans, and nuts, Eddie always had a portion of animal protein with his supper. But what and how much he consumed differed from the diets of many in this country. To begin with, he usually ate fish, typically steamed sea bass, which he enjoyed the most. For variety, chicken was occasionally on the menu, boiled and served without its skin. Red meats were the least likely to make it to his plate and, when eaten, were cut up into small pieces and mixed with vegetables or rice. For my dad, the animal protein was not the star of the dining experience. Instead, it played an equal or secondary role to the rest of the foods, complementing them. This resulted in him eating smaller, healthier amounts of animal products.

If we look at what Eddie ate—not forgetting that he loved his snacks—it's obvious there is really nothing exceptional about his food choices. Yes, it was overall healthy, similar in many ways to the Mediterranean diet: plenty of vegetables, fruits, legumes, nuts, and fish, with small amounts of red meats. But there was something else besides his meal choices that made his eating good for his health and longevity— something very simple but essential.

LIVING LONGER STARTS WITH YOUR BODY WEIGHT

When I think about how long Eddie lived, I recognize that maintaining a healthy body weight was one of the most important things he did to become a centenarian. Staying physically active helped, but his eating was the key. It prevented him from becoming overweight, a condition that has been shown to take years off life expectancy.

In America, excess body weight is one of the most serious health problems because of its high prevalence and increased risk for medical conditions such as heart disease, cancer, and diabetes—all leading causes of death. If you have a significant amount of excess weight, losing it is one of the most important steps you can take toward a healthier, longer life.

Losing excess weight can do the following:
- decrease your risk of heart disease and strokes
- reduce your chances of cancer
- prevent type 2 diabetes
- lower your blood pressure
- improve your cholesterol profile and reduce blood triglyceride (fat) levels
- decrease your risk of nonalcoholic fatty liver disease (presently the most common chronic liver condition in the United States)
- reduce the risk and severity of sleep apnea
- prevent arthritis and lessen joint pain
- make it easier for you to exercise (which can improve your health even more)

So, how do you achieve and stay at a healthy body weight that increases your chances of living to one hundred? Let's take an in-depth look at the factors that determine whether you lose, maintain, or gain weight.

A SIMPLE ENGINEERING APPROACH TO WEIGHT MANAGEMENT

Weight management is a frustrating and confusing subject for many. It's fraught with numerous misconceptions. You hear them all the time:

- "Skinny people have a higher metabolism and that's why they're so thin."
- "Eat healthier food and you will definitely lose weight."
- "Carbohydrates are unhealthy and cause obesity."

To understand how to effectively take control of your weight, you need to realize why these statements are not always true.

In college, I studied chemical engineering because of my fondness for chemistry and math. Chemical engineering encompasses these disciplines, along with physics and biology. Throughout my years as a physician and a health enthusiast, my training as an engineer has helped me better understand the intricate processes of the human body. The knowledge of some simple engineering concepts can do the same for you.

In order to comprehend the factors that determine how much you weigh, you need to appreciate the first law of thermodynamics. Initially proposed over a century and a half ago, it's a beautiful law—simple, elegant, and powerful. It is usually applied to situations involving nonliving things, such as the conversion of gasoline's chemical energy into the mechanical energy that powers a car. But this rule is universal and applicable to all things, including the living. Life is an inexplicable miracle, but all its physiological processes that keep us alive can ultimately be explained by scientific principles.

The first law of thermodynamics states that energy cannot be created or destroyed, that energy must be conserved. Let's translate this into more user-friendly terms by replacing the word "energy" with "calories." As we know, calories are present in the food we eat, and we burn them off through our metabolism and activities; calories are, in fact, units of energy. With this substitution, the law now reads as "calories cannot be created or destroyed, that calories must be preserved."

What does this mean? It tells you that if you eat more calories than your body utilizes, the extra calories must be preserved or saved. The body does this by storing the excess energy, usually as fat. Conversely, if you eat fewer calories than you utilize, the extra calories you burn off must be supplied by the body, which breaks down fat, muscle, or other tissues to release this energy.

The movement of calories through the body may be visualized with a simple engineering application called a flow diagram. We will use this diagram to examine the determinants of body weight, which can help you to understand any weight management problem. For those who are not science-oriented, please don't be intimidated—you'll see that it's not that complicated at all!

CALORIES FLOW IN AND OUT

The caloric flow diagram is merely an illustration of how calories enter and exit the body. Your body can be represented as a box in the center of the diagram. On the left-hand side is the "in" stream, which represents the calories coming into your body. On the right-hand side is the "out" stream, representing the calories leaving your body.

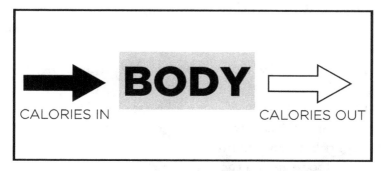

BASIC CALORIC FLOW DIAGRAM

The Input Stream: Only One Way In

On the input side, there is only one possible source of calories: the food you eat. When I use the word "food," I also mean drinks, such as soft drinks or alcohol. In a typical American adult's diet, 50 percent of calories come from carbohydrates, 15 percent from protein, and 35 percent from fats.

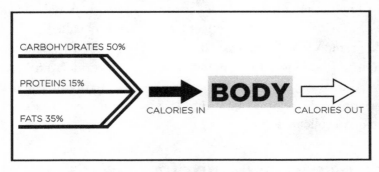

TYPICAL U.S. ADULT DIET MACRONUTRIENT INPUT

The Output Stream: Not One, but Three Possible Ways Out

While there is only one way to take in calories, there are three ways calories can leave your body: through metabolism at rest (basal metabolic rate), through physical activity, and through breaking down and processing what you eat (thermic effect of food).

In other words, you burn calories simply by existing, moving your body, and digesting your food.

On average, the basal metabolic rate makes up 60 to 75 percent of total energy expenditure, while physical activities contribute an additional 15 to 30 percent, and thermic effect of food supplies the final 10 percent. It is important to emphasize that these three output streams are the only means

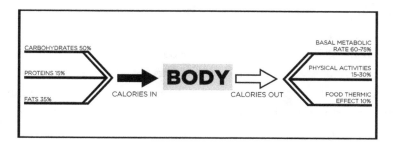

OUTPUT STREAM COMPONENTS

by which you can increase your caloric expenditure to lose weight. Recognizing the contribution of each output, as well as your ability to change them, is fundamental to effectively managing your body weight.

Basal Metabolic Rate (BMR): Your Stubborn Metabolism

You probably already know that increasing your metabolism will help you burn off more calories. But is it really possible to alter metabolism? Can it actually be raised by dieting, taking supplements, or exercising? And what does genetics have to do with it? Let's investigate some facts about metabolism and whether it can be manipulated to help you lose weight.

When most people talk about metabolism, they are essentially referring to the basal metabolic rate (BMR). This is a measurement of how many calories you burn per day to keep your basic life functions intact while at rest. These functions include breathing and blood circulation, cell and tissue repair, and maintenance of physiological processes, such as body temperature regulation. BMR typically makes up most of your total daily caloric output and usually accounts for more than twice the calories burned with physical activity. The four most metabolically demanding organs—the brain, heart, liver, and kidneys—account for over 70 percent of resting metabolism. These organs, by the way, make up only 8 percent of your body weight.

Your BMR is determined by a broad range of factors, including your age, sex, genetics, weight, and body composition. If you are young, male, or lean (i.e., you have a greater muscle-to-fat ratio), you are more likely to have a higher metabolism. Genetically, our BMRs can differ, but rarely by more than a few hundred calories per day. This is good news. It's not an insignificant number of calories, but fortunately it's not enough to be the sole cause of obesity. You are not destined to be overweight because of the metabolism given to you by your genes.

Body weight is a major determinant of BMR, but the relationship between the two is often confused. There is a common misconception that skinny people are skinnier because they have higher metabolic rates and heavy people are heavier because they have lower rates, but both beliefs are incorrect. The reality is that if you weigh less, you will likely have a decreased metabolic rate, and if you weigh more, you will likely have an increased rate. Why is this so?

Let's use a trick that I often apply when trying to figure out an engineering problem. I simply exaggerate one of the variables to clarify the issue.

Say you triple your weight. Now you have three times as much body mass to keep alive. Do you think you need more or less energy to maintain the physiological functions of all this additional living tissue? Clearly, a larger amount of energy or calories are required to sustain the increased body mass, and so your resting metabolism is greater when you weigh more. The same thinking applies when you weigh less. If you lose most of your body weight, you have far less energy-consuming tissue to support and therefore a lower BMR. So, in actuality, skinnier people possess a lower or "slower" metabolism and heavier people a higher or "faster" rate. Scientific measurements have confirmed this to be true. In fact, research shows that severely obese people can have metabolic rates that are more than 50 percent greater than those of people who have a normal weight.

At best, trying to manipulate your metabolism to manage your weight is a difficult proposition. Your metabolism is stubborn. It's not easy to change. The truth is that most of the factors that determine BMR—age, sex, and genetics—are beyond your control.

You can try to raise your metabolism by improving your body composition, but a large increase in the muscle-to-fat ratio is required before there is any meaningful elevation of BMR. The main calorie-burning benefit of obtaining a leaner body with additional muscle doesn't come from raising your resting metabolism rate, but from all the calories that must be expended to get, maintain, and use this leaner physique.

LET'S DO THE MATH

Here's why it's difficult to significantly raise your metabolism by improving your body composition. The caloric expenditure for a pound of resting muscle is six calories per day; for a pound of fat, it's two calories per day. So if, for example, you are able to put on ten pounds of muscle, your BMR increases by sixty calories. At the same time, if you are able to lose ten pounds of fat, your BMR decreases by twenty calories. With this improvement in body composition, the difference in resting metabolism is therefore only an additional forty calories per day—not an impressive amount.

What is impressive, though, is all the calories that are burned through exercising to achieve and keep up this change in body composition.

Afterburn—the continuous elevation of metabolism after exercising—does exist, but only following intense, sustained aerobic activities. Moreover, studies show that the effects of afterburn are limited: you only lose a fraction of the calories that you would otherwise burn from the actual workout. Weight is not lost due to any major changes in metabolism, but from performing the exercises themselves.

There are many claims that certain foods, spices, or supplements will sufficiently boost your metabolism so that you will effortlessly lose weight. Imagine if this were true. It would be the holy grail of weight loss solutions: you can eat as much as you want, you don't need to be physically active, and you will still burn off pounds of body mass because of your higher metabolism. Unfortunately, there is nothing you can eat that has been safely and scientifically proven to substantially raise your metabolism for weight loss purposes.

In summary, it is difficult to significantly increase your metabolism. Attempts to alter it are not the best means to lose weight.

Physical Activities: The Most Changeable Component of the Output Stream

In the next chapter, you'll learn about Eddie's active lifestyle. He easily expended hundreds of extra calories every day by constantly moving his body at work and at home. This high level of activity helped him to stay lean and healthy throughout his life.

Typically, 15 to 30 percent of the total calories you use daily are from physical activity, but this contribution to the output stream can vary tremendously. Calories burned by elite endurance athletes exercising during times of competitive training can easily exceed those consumed by their metabolism. It's even been said that the training regimens of some

Olympians are so extreme that these participants must eat close to ten thousand calories per day just to maintain their competition body weight.

How many calories you utilize during your activities depends on the intensity and duration of the movements, as well as how much you weigh. You can use metabolic equivalent of task (MET) values to help estimate how many calories you burn with a particular action. Think of MET as a measurement of the caloric intensity of a physical activity. It is based on oxygen consumption and is expressed as energy utilized per kilogram of body weight per hour. MET of one is the amount of energy your body uses while sitting at rest. Compared to sitting still, walking slowly consumes twice the number of calories, and so it has a MET of two. Vigorously jumping rope burns ten times the amount of calories as sitting and has a MET of ten, and so on. There are extensive lists of MET values online—a quick search should provide the numbers you need. To calculate the number of calories you burn for any activity, you simply multiply its MET value by your weight in kilograms and then by the number of hours you perform the movement.

It is important for you to realize that the physical activity stream is the most changeable factor on the output side. For those needing to lose only a small or moderate amount of weight, increased physical activity may be all that is necessary.

Thermic Effect of Food: Limited Effect on Calories Burned

Calories are needed to release the energy from the foods you eat. The thermic effect of food refers to the calories expended to digest and absorb what you consume. Protein requires your body to do the most work, costing 20 to 30 percent of its calories. So, if you eat one hundred calories of protein, your body will burn approximately twenty-five calories to process it. Carbohydrates and fats both have a significantly lower thermic effect—about 10 percent for carbs and only 5 percent or less for fats. Overall, the average American diet has a thermic effect of 10 percent of the calories eaten.

Some of you may be thinking, "If that many more calories are burned processing protein, why not just eat a mostly protein diet to lose weight?" In terms of numbers, this makes sense, but the problem is that it would be unhealthy to do so. Eating too much protein may deprive your body of other nutrients and is associated with increased risk of cardiovascular disease, cancer, and kidney damage. In fact, there is a recommended upper limit of safe protein intake for most healthy, normal-weight individuals, which is about 30 percent of your total calories consumed. How much protein you can safely eat depends on a number of factors including your age, bodyweight, activity level, and medical history. Consult with your doctor before changing the amount of protein you consume.

Presently, an average American adult eats a diet that is 15 percent protein by calories. You can increase your food-processing calories by eating more protein, but the effect is limited if you stay within the recommended guidelines for safe consumption. Increasing protein consumption is not the best means to lose weight.

LET'S DO THE MATH

For a two-thousand-calorie diet, doubling protein intake from 15 to 30 percent would only result in an increased energy expenditure of sixty-six calories, at best. Let's break down why. A two-thousand-calorie meal plan that is 15 percent protein contains three hundred calories of this macronutrient; double the protein content to 30 percent and it's six hundred calories. This means that three hundred additional calories of protein are replacing three hundred calories of carbohydrates or fats. With carbohydrates, the net difference in thermic effect is 25 percent (protein's thermic effect) minus 10 percent (carbohydrate's thermic effect). That's an increase in thermic effect of only 15 percent. Thus, replacing three hundred calories of carbohydrates with protein would only result in forty-five extra calories (15 percent of three hundred) expended to process the higher-protein diet. With fats—assuming a thermic effect of 3 percent—only sixty-six more calories are utilized. Thus, the best-case scenario you can hope for by increasing your protein intake within recommended limits is sixty-six calories. (For those of you who measure protein intake by grams, there are four calories in one gram of protein. So three hundred and six hundred calories of protein would respectively equal 75 and 150 grams of protein.)

THE SCIENTIFIC TRUTH ABOUT DIETS

You can apply the law of conservation of calories and the caloric flow diagram to help you think through different weight-management scenarios. Any diet, exercise plan, or other method you choose to lose weight must work by either decreasing the number of calories you ingest or by increasing the number of calories you burn. Let's look at dieting, the most common way we try to manage our weight.

There are hundreds of diets out there—food diets, fasting diets, diets that tell you to eat just one big meal or multiple small meals a day, and even a diet that tells you to wear blue-tinted glasses when dining. (Yes, this diet does exist!) None of them will appreciably raise the calories you burn through metabolism, physical activity, or food thermic effect. Therefore, they can only work to drop your body weight if they somehow cut the number of calories you eat. This is just the first law of thermodynamics at work.

The caloric flow diagram tells us that the body doesn't distinguish whether the calories are all eaten at one meal or over the course of ten meals. It doesn't recognize whether the calories are ingested early in the day, later in the day, or spread throughout the day. And whether the calories come from a piece of broccoli or from a doughnut is unimportant. A calorie is a calorie in the world of thermodynamics.

Ultimately, what matters for your body weight is the difference between calories in and calories out. That is why the Japanese population can seemingly eat lots of rice and carbohydrates without becoming obese or overweight. The secret is this: although they eat a high *percentage* of this nutrient group, the actual number of carbohydrate calories that they consume is not excessive. In short, their total caloric intake is low enough to prevent weight gain.

This, too, is how Eddie stayed lean. While he did eat rice with many of his lunches and dinners, it was, at most, a moderate amount. Moreover, his snacking was limited. I would estimate that he took in two hundred to three hundred calories per day from his treats. Typically, he had half a can of soda, a few Social Tea cookies, and either a small piece of dark chocolate or half a handful of chips. He didn't overeat his rice and snacks—his total calories eaten didn't exceed the calories his body burned.

A calorie is a calorie: this is why eating the healthiest foods may still result in unhealthy weight gain. It's simply because excess calories, regardless of their food source, will be conserved by the body. When you appreciate the first law of thermodynamics, you realize that eating for good health is not just about *what* you eat, but also about *how much* you eat.

Now, most diets may help you lose weight for a while because you can reduce the number of calories consumed. Some plans specifically tell you to eat less food, while others do so indirectly. For example, time-restricted eating programs may drop calories because they allow meals only during set hours, thus eliminating all-day eating and snacking. High-fiber diets can have you eating less by decreasing your body's production of hunger hormones. And wearing blue-tinted glasses during meals will cut down your calories because how much blue-colored foods do you want to eat? Whatever the means, the essential reason these diets work is that you take in fewer calories.

So, if diets work, why not just endlessly follow them to maintain a lower body weight? Because almost all diets will fail—statistically, over 95 percent fail within a year or two. They're just too restrictive and difficult to sustain. A change in eating habits that is lifestyle friendly is a more viable long-term solution for success.

PORTION CONTROL WORKS

Eddie never dieted, and he never thought about calories. He didn't need to because he had a healthy eating practice that kept him lean. It came from his upbringing in a poor family that had to divide among themselves whatever sustenance they could collect for the day. To start off the meal, each family member would take only small portions of what was available. This was to ensure that everyone had something on their plate. Then they would eat slowly to enjoy the food and come back for an additional serving, if any food was left over.

This way of eating became Eddie's version of portion control, which he unwittingly practiced all his life. He never started his meals with a full bowl of rice and a plate loaded with food—it was always a bowl of rice that was half-filled and a small amount of food. He would then take his time eating and later come back for more, if he still felt hungry. With this style of eating, he seldom overindulged.

Whatever methods you employ to decrease the size of your portions—using smaller dinnerware, reducing serving sizes, or simply eating like Eddie—limiting your portions may be the best long-term solution to maintaining a healthy body weight. Portion control is not as trendy as the latest fad diet, but it is practical, effective, and, most importantly, easy to sustain. There is no elimination of food groups, no unrealistic eating schedules, and no new cooking methods. You can incorporate portion control immediately into your lifestyle, and with fewer calories coming in, your body must follow the first law of thermodynamics, and you will lose weight.

ADDITIONAL HEALTHY EATING HABITS

Drinking Tea

While it's true that Eddie had a daily soda, he would also consume three to four cups of tea a day. When he was younger, he favored green teas, but he changed his taste to black teas by the time he reached his senior years. These drinks contain polyphenol compounds with antioxidant properties and have been associated with a decreased risk of heart disease, cancer, and diabetes.

Another important benefit of tea is that a plain cup of it is usually only a few calories. Just imagine if Eddie hadn't drunk tea and instead had consumed three to four additional glasses of soda each day. If he had, I doubt that he would have stayed lean and lived to be a centenarian. Drinking tea can reduce your caloric intake if it replaces your high-calorie beverages. For those who need to lose only a few pounds, this alone may get you to the weight you want.

Cutting Off the Burnt Pieces of Meat

Eddie dined on red meats sparingly. When he did eat them, he would cut away the fat and the burnt parts. The benefits of eating less fat from meats included consuming less choles-terol, which decreased the risk of heart disease. And when Eddie removed the charred portions, he reduced his chances of developing cancer.

Cooking meats at a very high temperature, such as by fry-ing, grilling, or barbecuing, can produce carcinogenic com-pounds such as heterocyclic amines. These substances can form in greater amounts when meats are overcooked or blackened. When Eddie removed the burnt parts of his steak, sausage, or chicken, he lowered his intake of these chemicals, which have been associated with malignancies of the colon, pancreas, and prostate.

Avoiding Spoiled Food

Growing up poor and often without much to eat, Eddie didn't like to waste food. But when food became old and spoiled, he didn't hesitate to throw it out. He would tell me that eating it wasn't worth the risk of getting sick.

Stale, rancid peanuts were an important example. He loved to eat peanuts, but when any one of them tasted bad or just didn't taste right, he discarded them. He was lucky that he did. Rancid peanuts produce aflatoxin, a known potent carcinogen that contributes to tens of thousands of liver cancers around the world each year.

Limiting Chemicals and Other Contaminants in Food

Eddie always preferred to dine on natural food. By avoiding canned and packaged meals, he reduced his consumption of potentially harmful preservatives. But eating natural didn't mean he wasn't exposed to other chemicals in his food. Pesticide residue can remain on fresh fruits and vegetables. My dad was very aware of this, thanks to his years of working on a farm when he arrived in the United States. This knowledge motivated him to wash his produce thoroughly before it was served or cooked.

To clean his fruits and vegetables, Eddie frequently used salt water. People in Asia have been using salt water as a general rinse for thousands of years. It is believed to have health-promoting properties, including antibacterial effects. He would soak the produce in salt water to kill the bacteria and then rinse repeatedly to wash away the chemicals and dirt.

THINGS TO KNOW FOR HEALTH AND LONGEVITY

1. There is no miracle longevity food; just eat a nutritious, well-balanced diet.
2. Maintaining a healthy body weight can add years to your life.
3. Ultimately, the first law of thermodynamics determines your weight.
4. Your metabolism is stubborn—it's difficult to change.
5. All diets can only work by reducing the number of calories you eat.
6. Eating for good health is not just about what you eat, but also about how much you eat.
7. Portion control is practical, effective, and, most importantly, easy to sustain.
8. Carbohydrates are not necessarily bad for you.
9. Eat proteins from healthy food sources such as fish, nuts, and legumes.
10. Limit your consumption of red meats.
11. Drink plenty of tea.
12. Cut off burnt pieces of meat.
13. Don't eat spoiled food, especially rancid peanuts.
14. Be aware of chemicals and other contaminants in your food.

NOTE

Diet and health are individual matters. Always consult a doctor about your specific needs before changing your diet.

ADDENDUM TO CHAPTER 1

Additional Applications of the Caloric Flow Diagram

The caloric flow diagram is not meant for you to plug in numbers and calculate how many fewer calories you need to eat, or how many more calories you must expend, to get to the weight you desire. First of all, numerous studies have shown that it is difficult to accurately count the number of calories eaten with meals or to estimate the calories used during physical activities. People consistently underestimate the food calories they ingest and overestimate the calories they burn. Also, obtaining an accurate BMR for the diagram would involve complex testing with respiratory gas analysis under strict resting and fasting conditions. Online BMR calculators are only estimates, which are limited in their accuracy because they don't take into account your actual body composition and cannot correct for genetic variability. They are based only on your age, height, weight, and sex.

So, what else can the caloric flow diagram do? It can help you visualize specific weight problems so that you can better understand how to manage them. Let's apply the diagram to a couple of scenarios: (1) what to do about gaining unwanted weight as we grow older and (2) how best to lose weight when we are significantly overweight.

YOU DON'T HAVE TO GAIN WEIGHT WITH AGING

Many of us collect extra pounds as we approach our middle-age years. Why does this happen and what can we do about it? The caloric flow diagram can provide guidance.

Let's begin by examining how our metabolism changes as we age. Starting in our late teens or early twenties, our organ systems begin to burn fewer calories (remember that the brain, heart, liver, and kidneys alone account for over 70 percent of BMR). We also start to lose muscle tissue—approximately 3 to 5 percent per decade after the age of thirty. By the time we reach seventy years of age, we may have lost half our muscle mass. Both of these factors will progressively decrease our metabolism from our mid-twenties onward.

Physical activity levels also typically fall as we get older. Most of us slow down and don't move around as much, and thus the calories we burn in the activity stream can drop significantly.

When we look at a typical aging caloric flow diagram, we see that the BMR and physical activities streams are decreased. It is obvious that, with these changes, if we continue to eat the same number of calories as we did when we were younger, we will have extra calories to conserve and will gain weight.

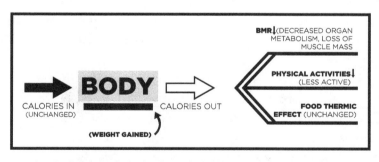

TYPICAL AGING CALORIC FLOW DIAGRAM

So, what can you do about putting on excess weight as you get older? Do what Eddie did. As he aged, he could do nothing about the naturally slowing metabolism of his internal organs, but he minimized his drop in BMR by maintaining his muscle mass. His daily work and home duties involved plenty of resistance movements, which slowed the loss of muscle. These responsibilities, along with his lifestyle, which involved always moving and never sitting too long, also kept up the calories he utilized in the activity stream. All of this limited the decrease in the total number of calories his body burned.

On the input side, if Eddie consumed the same amount of food calories as he had when he was younger, he probably would have still gained weight. Instead, he ate a bit less as he aged to keep in caloric balance.

So, to combat gaining weight as you age, you can do three things: incorporate resistance activities or exercises to preserve muscle tissue, stay physically active, and, if necessary, reduce the number of calories you eat.

THE BEST WAY TO FIGHT OBESITY

Presently, 40 percent of Americans aged twenty and over are obese—nearly triple the incidence of obesity in this country over the past fifty years. By examining the caloric flow diagram, we can gain some important insights into this condition and how to manage it.

With obesity, BMR is substantially elevated due to the extra calories required to sustain the additional body mass. The calories used to break down and process food are also increased, and this change is proportional to the excess calories eaten. The physical activities stream is highly variable—it can be up, down, or unchanged. If activity levels can be sustained, more calories are burned with a higher body weight. But, for some of those who are overweight, moving about or exercising can be difficult because of limited mobility, thus lowering their activity calories.

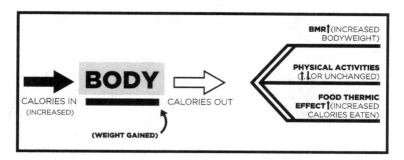

TYPICAL OVERWEIGHT CALORIC FLOW DIAGRAM

What we see with the flow diagram is an overall significant increase in calories leaving the body. Therefore, applying the first law of thermodynamics, the cause of obesity is clearly a higher number of calories entering the body, or simply overeating.

The amount of food consumed is the primary cause of obesity, and it's frequently the best solution to this condition. This is because raising the output calories enough to burn away all the excess calories taken in is difficult. The metabolic rate is already elevated and is difficult to raise further. Any attempt to increase the food thermic effect by eating a greater percentage of protein will result in only a small increase of calories burned off, as was shown previously. The only other output factor that can be manipulated is the activity stream, but the majority of people cannot exercise away a large amount of additional calories eaten.

It's not easy, but those who are obese can best achieve the necessary caloric deficit by restricting how much they eat. Proof that calorie reduction is an effective means to reduce weight in the severely overweight population is seen with bar- iatric surgery (weight loss surgery). The main mechanism of weight loss with these procedures is a restriction of the number of calories taken in by the body.

It is important to realize that as you lose weight, your metabolic rate will also drop accordingly—remember that your BMR is directly related to your body weight. This matters because, as your metabolism decreases with weight loss, you burn fewer resting calories. This means that you will have to *further* reduce your daily caloric intake to continue losing weight at the same pace. For example, if you needed to cut five hundred calories per day to lose the first ten pounds, you may now need to cut six hundred or more calories per day to lose the next ten pounds over the same time period.

Losing weight and maintaining the weight loss can be a challenge for many. So, if you're not able to do it alone, don't hesitate to seek medical or professional help to improve your chances of reaching a healthier body weight—your longevity depends on it.

THINGS TO KNOW FOR HEALTH AND LONGEVITY

15. The caloric flow diagram can help you manage your body weight.
16. As you age, incorporate resistance activities to preserve muscle mass, stay physically active, and, if necessary, reduce the number of calories you eat to avoid gaining excess weight.
17. If you are significantly overweight, eating fewer calories is often the best solution to losing the weight.

CHAPTER 2

GETTING ENOUGH PHYSICAL ACTIVITY WITHOUT EXERCISING

I watched my dad as he operated the old-fashioned commercial ironing press at the back of our family's dry-cleaning shop. With both arms extended above his head and his hands on the handle, he pulled down the machine's top plate onto the clothes he was pressing. At the same time, he stepped up onto one of the machine's control pedals—upward his body went for a foot or so, as steam was released onto the garment. He held this position for a few seconds before stepping back down to the floor. This maneuver was repeated eight or more hours a day, six days a week, until he retired at the age of seventy-five.

EDDIE'S ACTIVE LIFE

My dad had his first full-time job at the age of sixteen. To make money for his family, he worked as a deckhand on British cargo ships that picked up Chinese laborers from the Port of Shanghai. He would go out to sea for months at a time.

On the ships, he had a variety of assignments—everything from sweeping and mopping the decks, to washing the dishes in the kitchen, to shoveling coal in the boiler room. He told me he enjoyed his time out on the oceans, but it was hard, tiring labor. He continued this work until, one day in 1943, during World War II, his ship was unable to return to China due to increased maritime hostilities. So instead of navigating back to his homeland, the vessel docked in New York Harbor, where Eddie was dropped off at Ellis Island.

In America, Eddie soon found work as a farmhand in New Jersey. For a number of years, he tilled the soil, collected the crops, and tended to the chickens, cows, and horses. Eventually, he graduated to driving a farm truck to stores and vendors. Some of his responsibilities included loading and unloading heavy boxes and crates of produce and supplies. Again, it was hard labor, and he worked long hours, but it wasn't bad, he would tell me. He was happy to have a job, and the owners of the farms treated him well. After collecting enough money to go out on his own, Eddie bought a small laundromat in Chinatown, New York City, before moving up to a dry-cleaning business in New Jersey. He would work there for the next three decades, pressing clothes and managing the store.

Throughout his life, Eddie's jobs provided him with plenty of physical activity. After retiring, he continued to stay busy with household chores and home repairs. I remember a summer day when I helped my father fix an electric fan in the attic of the old house I grew up in. He was about eighty years old at the time.

In his detached garage, Eddie had a workshop where he kept his tools and electrical supplies. From this place, we had to walk to the house and up two flights of stairs to reach the attic. During our repair work, we had to go back to the garage repeatedly to get more equipment. I can remember making the trip four times over the next couple of hours—down the stairs, out to the garage, and then back into the house and up the stairs again. All that walking and stair climbing didn't bother or tire my dad one bit. For all his life, he was accustomed to moving his body.

THE BEST MEDICINE THERE IS

Eddie never once thought of the medical benefits he was getting from his work and activities, but they definitely helped to keep him fit and healthy. Without them, he would have been at an increased risk of developing heart disease, diabetes, and cancer, among other conditions. And if he hadn't used his body so much, I'm sure that he wouldn't have aged so well. Inactivity accelerates the aging process. The alterations that occur in the body with continuous sedentary living are similar to many of the changes that appear with old age: reduced physiological reserve of the heart, lungs, and other organs; diminished exercise capacity; and decreased muscle mass and strength with an increase in body fat. In fact, what we experience as we age is partly the result of our inactivity as we grow older.

Staying physically active like Eddie did is one of the best things you can do for good overall health. It benefits every part of your body, from your brain down to your toes. The use of your muscles to move about increases blood flow and oxygen delivery to all your organs and tissues. On a microscopic level, it rejuvenates your cells, preserving the functions of the cell's components. This includes the mitochondria, the powerhouse energy-producing intracellular structure that is essential for your quality of life, physical well-being, and longevity.

Increased physical activity can do the following:
- slow down the aging process and keep you looking young
- help with weight control and improve your body composition
- strengthen your heart, muscles, bones, and immune system
- lower your blood pressure and improve your cholesterol profile
- reduce your risk of diabetes, heart attack, stroke, and cancer
- improve your mood and sleep quality
- decrease your stress levels
- maintain your mobility and independence as you age and reduce your risk of dementia
- increase your life span and health span

Eddie's active lifestyle provided him with all these benefits. Many doctors say that physical activity is the best medicine there is for good health. It's also the closest thing we have to the fountain of youth.

WHY EXERCISING IS UNNECESSARY FOR SOME

In his 101 years of life, Eddie never exercised once. But when I think about him pressing clothes in the dry-cleaning shop—his hands reaching up and pulling down the plate of the ironing machine—the movements and contractions of the muscles in his arms, shoulders, and back remind me of a common calisthenics exercise, the pull-up. This action was coupled with what appeared to be another frequent workout maneuver, the leg step-up, as he lifted his right foot off the ground to apply pressure onto the elevated floor pedals of the apparatus.

If you'd watched Eddie at work, you would never have said that he was exercising. But dress him in athletic shorts and a T-shirt, and remake the drab old pressing machine into a shiny chrome exercise contraption, you would view these same movements as exercise. So, what exactly is the difference between physical activity and exercise, and does the body really know or care?

The distinction between what we call activity and what we call exercise lies in the intention behind the movements. Physical activity is any motion of the body involving the skeletal muscles that consumes energy. Lifting grocery bags, mopping the floors, and planting flowers are all considered activities. Exercise is a type of activity and is defined as a planned, organized, and repetitive movement with the goal of maintaining or improving physical fitness. Based on this definition, almost any activity can be considered exercise if it is structured and done for reasons of fitness—walking briskly, swimming laps, and dancing aerobically, for example. I guess if Eddie thought of his efforts at pressing clothes as a means to staying fit, it too could be considered exercise.

The distinction between the two doesn't matter to your body. Whether you are forced to climb multiple flights of stairs because of a broken elevator or choose to climb those same stairs for fitness reasons, the activity provides health benefits to your body.

For those of you who may not like to exercise, it's good to know that you don't have to—but you do need to live a physically active life. In fact, there is no scientific evidence that exercising is better for your health than an overall active lifestyle. Most of the populations from regions of the world where people live the longest are proof of this. They don't go to gyms to work out or seek activities to stay fit. Instead, like Eddie, they labor at their jobs and participate in daily household chores and tasks that involve using their bodies to push, pull, and lift things. An active way of life is sufficient for them to stay healthy. That said, some of us, because we don't move enough at our jobs or at home, will need to participate in activities with the specific intention of improving our fitness and health. In other words, some of us will have to exercise.

HOW MUCH ACTIVITY DO YOU ACTUALLY NEED?

The American Heart Association (AHA) recommends that people between the ages of eighteen and sixty-four get at least 150 minutes of moderate aerobic activity or seventy-five minutes of vigorous aerobic activity per week. Typical moderate activities are bicycling on a level road, playing doubles tennis, and light gardening. Common vigorous activities include running, hiking uphill, and playing basketball.

The AHA additionally recommends strength and resistance training, such as lifting weights, at least twice a week. The purpose of this type of activity is to maintain the mass and strength of both your muscles and bones. As you age, resistance exercises can improve your quality of life and prevent you from becoming frail, a condition that elevates your overall mortality risk.

STAND UP FOR YOUR HEALTH

Eddie didn't like to sit for too long. He loved to stand and took every opportunity to do so. If he was eating alone, it wasn't uncommon to find him on his feet for the entire meal, despite the empty chairs around him. And when he was retired and had the time to read for extended periods, he would frequently alternate between sitting and standing while perusing his newspapers, magazines, or books. This love of standing was present all through his life.

Unbeknownst to Eddie, this habit protected his health. It decreased the total number of hours he sat during the day and prevented him from sitting for long stretches of time without a break. Both excessive sitting and prolonged continuous sitting are detrimental to your physical well-being. Studies have shown that staying seated for over eight hours a day increases your chances of cardiovascular disease, dementia, and cancer. Moreover, continuously sitting for more than half an hour straight raises your mortality rate.

To minimize the negative health effects of sitting, you need to both limit the number of hours in this position and avoid stretches of uninterrupted sitting. This is regardless of your overall activity level—don't think that an hour of exercise or being otherwise active for the rest of the day will make up for unhealthy sitting habits.

For every thirty minutes of sitting, get up and move around for at least a minute or two. When you do rise from your chair, you don't need to run around or perform jumping jacks. Just do what Eddie did: stand up and walk around a bit. This alone can temporarily boost the circulation of blood through your body and reduce the risks from continuous sitting.

KEEP CLIMBING STAIRS

Even after becoming a centenarian, Eddie was able to climb stairs. Although his steps became slow and deliberate, climbing was no small feat. This activity, which many of us take for granted, involves the use of the largest muscle groups in the body and requires a sufficient amount of core strength and aerobic fitness. It helped to maintain his muscle mass and kept his heart strong in his later years. By itself, stair climbing can be a great exercise for staying fit and healthy at any age.

My dad maintained the ability to walk up the stairs throughout his life, thanks in part to an active lifestyle that kept him fit. But perhaps the most important reason that Eddie was still able to climb stairs at one hundred was simply because he never stopped doing so. For most of his life, it didn't matter if there were two, three, or more flights—he climbed them. Some people intentionally avoid stairs and thus, when they become seniors, walking up a flight or two becomes a difficult or impossible endeavor. As we grow older, we can use it or lose it when it comes to such activities.

Use the stairs. It's a great activity or exercise that can help keep you fit and healthy.

WALK BACKWARD TO KEEP MOVING FORWARD

On his hundredth birthday, Eddie showed off to me: he walked backward across his bedroom. It was a wonderful sight to behold. He was able to pull off this act because walking backward was an activity he often engaged in. Frequently when standing, he would take a few steps backward and then retrace the steps moving forward.

Walking backward makes your legs stronger by exercising those muscles in your lower extremities that are not used during normal ambulation. It improves your balance, agility, and flexibility—important factors that decrease your risk of falling, which is the leading cause of injury and accidental death in the elderly. It is also said to sharpen your mind because it challenges your brain to do something different.

All it takes is a routine of taking a step or two back while you are standing. Do this throughout your day, as Eddie did. You can also try dancing or tai chi. Both of these activities incorporate backward movements.

BE CONSCIOUS OF YOUR POSTURE

Eddie had no chronic knee, hip, or back pains, which so many people experience as they age. What did he do that helped him avoid these conditions?

Staying lean and being physically active helped. He had less body weight to cause continuous wear and tear on his body. His constant movements—especially resistance activities—strengthened the muscles, tendons, and ligaments that protected his joints. Also important, when he sat, stood, and walked, he did so with good posture. He kept his head up, his shoulders back, and his spine in proper alignment. This led to more efficient and coordinated muscle movements and less mechanical stress and damage to his skeletal system.

Our posture is the result of numerous muscles contracting in an attempt to keep our spine and joints in proper position. We maintain our posture without thinking and have been doing so since we were babies, when we learned how to counteract the effects of gravity to balance ourselves and move about. Eddie was fortunate to have naturally good posture; he never had to think about it. But for many of us, good posture does not come naturally. We need to be conscious of it and strive for correct posture to lessen our chances of developing future joint problems.

ESTABLISH A CONSISTENT SLEEPING ROUTINE

Eddie had good sleeping habits. He followed a nighttime

routine that he seldom deviated from—in bed by 11:00 p.m. and awake by 6:00 a.m. It didn't matter if it was a weekday or the weekend; he kept to this schedule. It was especially important for him to get good sleep because of how physically active he was during the day.

After my dad retired in his late seventies, he started to take afternoon naps. Initially, the naps were half an hour, but they increased to a couple of hours or more in the last few years of his life. The naps seemed to be a good thing. They rejuvenated Eddie, giving him additional energy for the rest of the day.

A routine of regular sleep and rest plays an important role in your overall health. This is when your body builds and repairs its tissues, strengthens its immune system, and regulates body hormones. It's also the time when your mind can recharge, improving your mood, memory, and mental productivity.

Insufficient and excessive sleep are both associated with an increased risk of many of the leading causes of morbidity and mortality, such as heart disease, stroke, and diabetes. Studies have shown that less than six hours of sleep a day is associated with an increased risk of death. The same is true if you sleep more than nine hours a day. That is why doctors recommend that adults get seven to eight hours of sleep a night to stay in good health.

THINGS TO KNOW FOR HEALTH AND LONGEVITY

18. Physical activity is the best medicine there is.
19. The body doesn't recognize the difference between activity and exercise.
20. You don't need to exercise if you are active enough in your daily life.
21. Get at least 150 minutes of moderate physical activity or 75 minutes of vigorous physical activity per week.
22. Make sure your activities include resistance movements.
23. Avoid sitting for over eight hours a day.
24. For every thirty minutes of continuous sitting, get up and move around for a minute or two.
25. Stand frequently for good health.
26. Don't avoid stairs; keep climbing them.
27. Walk backward for your mind and body.
28. Good posture is good for your joints.
29. Establish a consistent routine of sleeping seven to eight hours a night.

NOTE

Physical activity and health are individual matters. Always consult a doctor about your specific needs before increasing your activity level or starting any new exercise or exercise program.

CHAPTER 3

THREE PESSIMISTIC EXPECTATIONS TO MANAGE STRESS

As a child, Eddie occasionally walked by the British pastry shop in a Westernized part of Shanghai, at a time when the cosmopolitan city was known as "the Paris of the East" and "the New York of the West." He peered into the store's window and stared at all the breads, cakes, and cookies that were available to eat. He was amazed by the variety of treats on display.

When I first heard this story from my father, I asked him if this experience made him sad, as I knew he was too poor at the time to purchase any of the delicacies. "Never," he said. "It made me happy. I liked coming to the store and thinking about what each piece would taste like. I believed that one day I would not have to imagine—that, one day, I could eat such foods."

EDDIE'S PERSPECTIVE ON LIFE

Eddie always felt he was very fortunate in his life. He would repeatedly say to me, "I'm so lucky. I can't ask for more."

These feelings of good fortune existed despite a childhood that was devoid of steady meals, education, and healthcare. They remained during Eddie's separation from his family after he landed in America. And they continued regardless of the long, hard hours he endured when working. Despite these hardships, Eddie always felt blessed. Why was this so?

"How you see life is how you experience life," he used to say to me. "We all look at things differently. At times, we can choose to be happy when others are sad, and we can choose to be calm when others are troubled." It was his perspective on life and his perception of its events that kept my father content.

Expectations shape perception, and there were three expectations that Eddie lived by and taught me. He used these beliefs to successfully navigate this sometimes troublesome and uncertain world.

These were the three expectations Eddie believed in:

1. **Life is hard.** Expect difficult times, unexpected problems, and obstacles in your path. Expect to work hard to achieve what you desire.
2. **Life is not equal and fair.** Expect that some are born into or given advantages in life that you do not have. Expect that you will not always get what you think you deserve.
3. **Life does not owe you happiness.** Expect that happiness will not come to you without effort. Expect to find happiness by searching within yourself for what makes you happy.

At first glance, these convictions appear harsh, the thoughts of a glum pessimist. But from a lifetime of knowing my father, I understand that nothing could be further from the truth. He was quite the opposite—amazingly cheerful and optimistic, always looking at the positive side of life. But he understood that there were certain realities that he had to accept, including things that he couldn't change or control. Because he had these expectations, he was more psychologically prepared and less stressed by the challenges that confronted him. He expected that he had to overcome difficulties and work diligently to succeed and arrive at a point in his life where, among other things, he could taste those treats that he had looked at so longingly through the pastry shop window as a child.

It should be noted that Eddie's expectations of difficult times didn't mean he had low expectations for his life. He always dreamed of having his own business one day. When he arrived in America, owning a business was a lofty goal for an uneducated laborer in a new country, speaking a different language. But he believed that it was possible, and he achieved it.

MENTAL STRESS HURTS THE BODY

Eddie's perspective on life enabled him to cope well with stress and was an important contributor to his good health and longevity. The ability to cope with stress is a common trait found in centenarians, and that's because mental stress is not just in your head.

When your mind is stressed, it causes physiological changes in your body. Adrenaline (epinephrine) is released early in the stress response. It's the "fight or flight" hormone that prepares the body to handle what is causing the tension. In past times, it was a necessary survival response that protected us from physical dangers, such as predators. Today, the response still remains and can be triggered by anything you perceive as stressful.

Adrenaline is responsible for the initial symptoms you may experience when you are anxious—an increase in heart rate, shaking, and jittery feelings, for example. Cortisol, a type of steroid produced by the body, is also released into the bloodstream. It's an essential chemical needed for the maintenance of good health, but, like many other substances, too much of it is harmful. Increased cortisol levels can raise blood pressure, decrease immune response, and impair cognitive function.

Here's how frequent triggering of the stress response can affect the major systems of the body:
- Circulatory—faster heart rate; higher blood pressure; increased risk of heart attack, arrhythmia, and stroke
- Respiratory—rapid respiratory rate, difficulty breathing, shortness of breath
- Digestive—increased stomach acid production; ulcers, abdominal bloating and discomfort; changes in bowel habits
- Nervous—headaches, difficulty sleeping, increased risk of dementia
- Endocrine—worsening of diabetes, disruption of menstrual cycle
- Immune—suppression of immune function, increased risk of infections
- Muscular—muscular tension; shoulder, neck, and back pain
- Integumentary (skin)—worsening of eczema and psoriasis, thinning or loss of hair
- Reproductive—infertility, low sex drive, erectile dysfunction

Besides these detrimental effects, mental stress also damages your DNA. It shortens telomeres, the end sections of your chromosomes, which protect your genetic code and assist in proper chromosome replication. Shorter telomeres are associated with the aging of cells and an increased risk of cancer.

STRESSORS DON'T HAVE TO PRODUCE STRESS

When I worked with Eddie on repairing the attic fan in our old house, it was supposed to be a simple job. But as the work progressed, it soon became evident that the task wasn't going to be easy. It evolved into quite a complicated endeavor, requiring much more time than anticipated and multiple trips out to the garage for additional tools and supplies. It could have been frustrating for my dad, but this potential mental stressor didn't faze him at all.

A stressor is a situation, event, or any other thing that causes stress in an individual. Your perception of the stressor plays an important role in how much mental pressure you feel. Giving a speech in front of a large audience is a common stressor. This may be something you try to avoid at all costs because you perceive it to be terrifying. You may even feel nauseous with your heart pounding, muscles tensing, and palms sweating just from thinking about it. For others, it's a welcomed opportunity to present their thoughts, and it produces little or no stress. It's the same stressor, but with vastly different physiological responses because of differing perceptions.

How you respond to everyday stressors can influence your mental and physical health. Stressors don't necessarily have to produce stress.

Change your reaction to a stressor by asking yourself
the following questions:
- Is it even worth stressing about?
- Is your perception of the stressor accurate?
- If possible, can you alter your perception?
- Is the stress from unrealistic expectations?
- If possible, can you alter your expectations?

Altering your perception of daily stressors is an important technique to avoid excessive triggering of the stress response. This can help you reduce the overall amount of mental pressure in your life.

CHARACTER TRAITS THAT IMPROVE HEALTH

Along with his positive perspective on life, Eddie also possessed character traits that enhanced his health. These attributes have been shown in numerous studies to increase happiness, decrease anxiety, and improve our overall physical well-being. A few traits stand out in my mind that also describe well the person that my dad was. When I think about the times I spent with him, so many of his words and actions clearly reflect these qualities.

Humility

"I did nothing special."

When Eddie turned one hundred years old, I presented him with a letter from the White House, signed by the president. It wished him a happy hundredth birthday. He examined the paper, carefully reading and rereading the words.

Unbeknownst to him, it was a form letter, but I didn't tell him so.

"It's from the president," I said with a smile. "The president of the United States. He's wishing you a happy birthday!"

I could see the confusion on his face. He was thinking, "Why would someone so important be sending me birthday wishes?" Another minute passed while he continued to scrutinize the letter. He then said, "I did nothing special. I only lived a long life."

Making it to his hundredth birthday was nothing exceptional to Eddie, despite all the congratulations from family, friends, and even the president. In actuality, it's quite an accomplishment, considering the fact that only a fraction of 1 percent of the men born in 1916 lived to be centenarians. But my dad didn't believe he deserved any special praise for it. "I didn't try to live so long; it just happened," he would also say.

This response to the letter didn't surprise me because Eddie had always been a humble person. The humility he possessed produced a sense of peace in his heart and mind. He didn't need to prove his worth; he accepted who he was. It also nurtured in him a compassion for his fellow men and women. He valued other people, and he treated everyone he encountered with respect. In return, they showed him respect, which made Eddie feel good about himself and his life.

Gratitude

"Thank you, thank you, thank you."

During Eddie's early years in China, neighbors helped his family by providing food and lending money when times were especially lean. He didn't know how they would have survived without this help.

These acts of kindness left a lasting impression on my father; he was forever grateful for the goodness he received from people. He would show his appreciation of their thoughtfulness by saying, "Thank you, thank you, thank you."

Gratitude made Eddie feel that the world was a place where people cared and were willing to help one another. This recognition of people's goodwill and his appreciation for what he had in life created positive emotions that enhanced his health. He believed that he was fortunate and blessed.

When my dad wanted to show his gratitude, he would purposely say "thank you" three times in succession. This repetition mirrored the Chinese custom of bowing three times to pay respect. "Thank you, thank you, thank you" was Eddie's way of simultaneously giving thanks and symbolically offering three bows to show his sincere gratitude for what he had received.

Empathy

"Think how they feel."

In my youth, I helped with the family's dry-cleaning business. I worked at the front of the shop, managing customers who dropped off and picked up their garments. When I started, my dad had a talk with me about the business. He told me that some people might not be able to pay their bills, but they still needed their clothes.

"Think how they feel," he said. "They would pay if they could, but life must be hard for them at this time. Let them have their clothes and ask that they pay later, whenever they can."

Eddie empathized with people facing difficulties in their lives. He remembered when he was in their shoes, and he felt their pain. Empathizing with what people were going through inspired my dad to help. The act of helping others gave Eddie's life more meaning, and it made him feel good that he could be of assistance.

Curiosity

"Because there is so much to learn."

A few months after my father's hundredth birthday, I walked into his room and there he was, standing next to his table, reading his newspaper—a familiar sight. My dad became an avid reader after he retired, consuming papers, magazines, and books for hours on end, every day.

That afternoon, I asked, "Dad, you're one hundred years old. Why do you still read so much?"

He put his newspaper down, looked at me, and said without hesitation, "Because there is so much to learn."

Eddie's curiosity was a great trait for him to have, especially as he grew older, because it kept his mind busy. In his later years, I could still see the excitement on his face when he discovered something new. His interest in a variety of subjects and his continuous desire to learn gave him happiness and prompted him to stay active and engaged in life.

HAVING A PURPOSE IN LIFE MOTIVATES YOU TO LIVE

When friends visited my home, Eddie would frequently come out to greet them, even after he became a centenarian. He would smile, say his hellos, and make conversation for a few minutes before returning to his bedroom. This simple, welcoming act warmed the hearts of many.

Contributing to the welfare of the family was Eddie's main purpose in life. It made him feel useful—a feeling he treasured. His greetings when company arrived were an example of this. He believed that guests should be greeted by all the household members, and he happily did his part.

Studies have shown that having a purpose in life leads to better health and decreased mortality. A purpose can make life more fulfilling, as it adds meaning to your existence. In old age, it becomes especially important because that purpose can provide the energy to get you up in the morning and keep you moving forward throughout the day. In fact, it gave Eddie the courage, strength, and will to overcome a life-threatening condition he faced in the last decade of his life.

KEEP CLOSE, NURTURING RELATIONSHIPS TO STRENGTHEN YOUR HEALTH

When my daughters were infants, my father taught them a special hello. He would hold out his index finger and my girls would hold out theirs. Both would reach out until their fingers touched. This simple action was a ritual for the rest of their lives and came to symbolize their love for one another. As adults, my daughters still used it whenever they greeted him. When he was bedridden for a year from a serious illness, and it was difficult to hug him, this touching of the fingers was adopted by the rest of the family. It was a small gesture, but it meant a lot to my dad and his loved ones.

Eddie's bond with his family undoubtedly contributed to him reaching his final years. It gave him a reason to live and fight on when he was sick. When you are connected with people who support you emotionally, you can weather disease and stressful times more effectively. Studies have shown that close, nurturing relationships strengthen your immune system and can improve your health, increase your longevity, and even decrease your risk of dementia.

IT'S IMPORTANT TO TAKE A BREAK
FROM WORK AND STRESS

Even when Eddie was working long hours running his shop, he would always find time to unwind. One of his favorite activities to help him relax was painting, which he would do a couple times a week. His artworks were mostly of the ocean, perhaps because of all the years he spent out at sea. "I'm not very good at painting, but it's fun," he would say. To Eddie, the fun part was all that mattered.

Like Eddie, you need to give your mind and body a chance to take a breather from all the stressors in your life. These breaks help to combat the negative physiological effects of stress. They can lower your blood pressure and heart rate and normalize your cortisol levels. It's also an opportunity for you to reset yourself—to reorganize and re-energize. These respites from stress are essential for continued good health.

You can exercise to de-stress; this may include workouts that purposefully relax the mind, such as yoga or tai chi. You can meditate, practice breathing techniques, or even try biofeedback to reduce mental tension. Or you can do your own thing, such as listening to music, taking walks in nature, or painting the ocean. It's important that you find an activity that works for you and make the time for it.

During stressful periods, you must also still take good care of your body: eat healthy, stay physically active, and get enough sleep. Despite your efforts, if you constantly feel overwhelmed and out of control or if the psychological strain interferes with essential day-to-day activities of your life, you should seek help from a mental health professional.

THINGS TO KNOW FOR HEALTH AND LONGEVITY

30. How you see life will influence how you experience it.
31. Mental stress can damage your physical health.
32. Your expectations shape your perceptions.
33. Identify and evaluate the stressors in your life.
34. Changing your perception of a stressor can reduce the amount of stress you experience.
35. Adopt character traits that improve your health.
36. Make sure you have a purpose in life.
37. Stay socially connected with people who support you emotionally.
38. Participate in stress-reducing activities.
39. Don't hesitate to seek help from a mental health professional.

CHAPTER 4

HABITS THAT CAN SHORTEN YOUR LIFE SPAN

I parked the car on the street in front of my parents' home. Off early from work at the hospital, I decided to pay them a visit. As I stepped onto the sidewalk, I heard my name.

"Hi Bill."

I looked around. I recognized the voice, but I didn't see my father.

"Bill, up here."

I turned my head to look up to the top of the house, and there he was, at ninety years old—my dad, standing on the roof.

EDDIE'S MOST UNHEALTHY HABIT

The habits you follow can determine how healthy you are and how long you live. There are habits that are good for you and others that are not. Overall, Eddie had many healthy habits. He ate a nutritionally balanced diet and didn't overeat, stayed physically active, and slept seven hours a night. But Eddie did have one very bad habit. Luckily, it didn't shorten his life.

Walking on the roof that day to find and repair a water leak was just one example of this habit. It was his tendency to engage in activities that qualify as risk-taking behaviors—activities that could result in bodily harm and even death. Despite whatever excuse he used, it wasn't safe to climb up onto the roof by himself at that age. And he did it regardless of an accident he had decades earlier, when he fell fifteen feet off a ladder and suffered injuries that landed him in the hospital.

Climbing up high wasn't the only risky behavior my dad was involved in during the later years of his life. In his nineties, it wasn't uncommon to find him, after a winter storm, walking outside, chipping ice off the car's windshield or shoveling the snow. For the very old, these are dangerous activities that can result in serious harm from a slip and fall or a heart attack from overexertion. We pleaded with him to stop, but he always had an explanation as to why it was okay. "It's just a little bit of ice on the ground," or, "It's not heavy snow," he would say.

His final risky act played out as I sat as a passenger in his car. He wanted to go to the supermarket and offered to drive. I remembered my dad as a safe driver, but it had been many years since I had sat in a car with him behind the wheel. I expected a nice easy ride on the local roads, but he surprised me. He drove onto a busy expressway, and for the next five minutes, I witnessed my dad weaving in and out of traffic, above the speed limit. Operating a vehicle like this is a risky behavior—regardless of the age of the driver. It endangered him and his passengers, as well as others on the road.

All these incidents finally convinced me to ask my parents to live in my home. Within half a year of the highway episode, they would sell their house, donate his car, and move in—no more working on the roof, shoveling snow, or driving for Eddie.

Risk-taking behaviors come in all forms. They can vary from texting while driving to not wearing a helmet while bicycling to using illicit drugs. Eddie believed that what he was doing was safe. Those who engage in these activities may believe the same too, but they must realize that it's not always so. Such behavior can present a real possibility for injury, illness, or even death. As a doctor, I have seen and treated the results of such actions and, sadly, know that the harm it caused was largely preventable.

SMOKING AND EXCESSIVE DRINKING
ARE MORE HARMFUL THAN YOU THINK

Fortunately for Eddie, he didn't smoke and he rarely drank. I doubt that he would have made it to his centenarian years if these habits had been part of his lifestyle. When he did consume alcohol, it was always a small amount and only for exceptional occasions, such as his hundredth birthday, when family and friends insisted on a toast.

I am sure you know that these behaviors are bad for you— that the lungs are damaged with smoking and the liver damaged with drinking. But the harm they inflict on the body is much more extensive. Both of these habits aggressively attack multiple organ systems and are associated with other dangers that you may not be aware of. Take, for example, how they interact with anesthesia.

When smokers wake up from a general anesthetic, it isn't a pretty sight—there are copious oral secretions, thick mucus from the lungs, and spitting and coughing upon awakening. It can be a mess. Smoking increases the risk of intraoperative pulmonary problems, such as poor air exchange and low blood oxygen levels. Alcohol abuse also raises the risk of anesthetic complications. Among other things, it can alter the metabolism and the required dosages of drugs, as well as causing cardiac and pulmonary instability during surgery.

While dealing with these physiological challenges in the surgical suite, I have also observed firsthand the visible anatomical changes that occur. Once-beautiful organs are distorted by years of abuse—lungs are dirtied, darkened, and deformed by multiple irregularly enlarged air spaces scattered throughout their structure, and cirrhotic livers, whose surfaces were once smooth and glistening, are now dulled, scarred, and filled with grotesque nodules.

SMOKING DISRUPTS THE PROCESS OF BREATHING

In the last few years of his life, Eddie called his body an old car and his heart a worn-out engine. Imagine, like Eddie did, the human body to be a machine, with its organ systems as different functional parts. This is a simplistic but helpful way to understand some basic anatomy and physiology. Just as the heart can be considered a pump (instead of an engine), the lungs can be thought of as a gas exchanging device. The swapping of gases occurs at the alveoli, the microscopic bubble-shaped air sacs that compose the lungs.

Carbon dioxide is a waste product of the metabolic reactions in your body. Your blood carries carbon dioxide to your lungs, so that it can be eliminated when you exhale. The exchange occurs through the tiny capillaries that pass next to the one-cell-thick walls of the alveoli—carbon dioxide is dropped off and oxygen is picked up by the blood. Smoking disrupts this process. It destroys the delicate walls of these air sacs and the surrounding capillaries. With fewer alveoli and capillaries remaining, the lungs' ability to exchange gases is impaired.

Smoking also induces an inflammatory reaction in the bronchial tree, the system of tubes that distributes the air you breathe from your trachea down to the alveoli. This results in an overabundance of mucus production and accumulation of debris in the bronchial airways, which increases the resistance to airflow within the lungs. The airway obstruction created by this process can further reduce the lungs' ability to oxygenate blood and breathe out carbon dioxide.

Another pulmonary consequence of smoking includes a greater risk of catching the flu and pneumonia. If a smoker contracts these illnesses, the condition is oftentimes more severe than in a nonsmoker. There are many reasons for this, including damaged lung anatomy, decreased ability to clear the airways, and suppressed body immune response. The result of these effects was seen in the recent COVID-19 pandemic—smokers had a higher probability of ICU admissions and deaths.

EXCESSIVE DRINKING DAMAGES OUR BODY'S MAIN CHEMICAL FACTORY

Think of your liver as your body's main chemical factory. Chemical factories manufacture, transform, and break down substances. Your liver does much the same things. It produces essential blood clotting factors and bile, which aids in the digestion of food. It metabolizes proteins, fats, and carbohydrates. And it takes apart, detoxifies, and removes many drugs and chemicals from your body. Your liver has all these vital functions, so you can see why keeping your liver healthy is important to your physical well-being.

Alcohol abuse is a major cause of chronic liver disease in the United States. Alcohol is directly toxic to your liver cells, and its breakdown product, acetaldehyde, is even more so. Excessive alcohol consumption can also damage the liver by altering fat metabolism. Abnormal amounts of fat accumulate in this organ because of drinking, and this may lead to hepatitis, cirrhosis, and even possible liver failure.

While a chronic alcoholic can present special challenges to an anesthesia provider, so too can the binge drinker who is acutely intoxicated. Alcohol is a drug (since it possesses physiological effects when introduced into the body) and can interact with anesthetic medications, heightening anesthesia's depressant effects on the heart, lungs, and brain. That is also why you should not mix alcohol with drugs, especially narcotics and sedatives: because life-threatening oversedation can readily occur.

IT'S NOT JUST THE LUNGS OF SMOKERS AND THE LIVERS OF DRINKERS

Even as a doctor, I was surprised at how much damage smoking and drinking inflict on the body. Smoking cigarettes raises your risk of heart attacks, strokes, and peripheral vascular disease (narrowing or blockage of blood vessels). In addition to an increased risk of lung cancer—which is the leading cause of cancer deaths—you increase the probability of many other malignancies. The list includes cancers of the pancreas, kidney, bladder, esophagus, stomach, and colon. Smoking's damage to the body is vast. Smoking is also associated with cataracts, osteoporosis, and infertility.

Besides these health issues, smoking is one of the worst habits you can have if you are concerned about your appearance as you age. It wrinkles and loosens your skin, grays and thins out your hair, and discolors your teeth and nails. If you want to look as young as possible for as long as possible, don't smoke.

Smokers may go to plastic surgeons when they want to reverse the visible signs of aging. Although smoking provides these doctors with additional patients, plastic surgeons disapprove of this habit more than all other surgeons. They don't like the fact that smoking impairs wound healing and increases the chances of postoperative infections. Because smoking decreases the oxygen content of the blood and restricts blood supply to the wound, it's more difficult for the incisions to heal. That is why smokers about to have plastic procedures are often instructed to refrain from the habit for weeks before and after their operations.

As with smoking, alcohol impacts many organs. It damages the brain, diminishing your cognitive abilities, such as memory. Other neurological conditions associated with drinking are ataxia (loss of coordination), peripheral nerve damage, and seizures. Alcohol weakens the heart, deteriorating the pumping action of this muscular structure, and this can lead to congestive heart failure. Digestive tract problems, such as chronic inflammation of the esophagus and stomach, are also common, with increased danger of ulcer formation. This can lead to serious gastrointestinal bleeding. Finally, not to be outdone by smoking, drinking raises your chances of liver, mouth, throat, esophageal, colon, and breast cancers.

IT CAN LAND YOU ON THE
OPERATING ROOM TABLE

You don't want to have surgery unless you have to—especially an emergency operation. Nonelective procedures are associated with increased surgical and anesthesia complication rates. Unfortunately, smoking and drinking increase the likelihood that you will land unexpectedly on an operating room table.

For smokers, operations are needed to resect pockets of infections in the lungs, reopen blocked arteries throughout the body, and amputate toes—and sometimes feet—when lower extremity revascularization operations fail or are not feasible. Drinkers require repairs of fractured bones from slips, falls, and car accidents while intoxicated. Additionally, there are endoscopies for the multiple gastrointestinal disorders brought on by alcohol. These include procedures to stop life-threatening bleeding from ulcers and esophageal varices (enlarged veins in your esophagus, frequently caused by cirrhosis).

QUIT—IT'S THE BEST THING YOU CAN DO FOR YOUR HEALTH

Quitting either one of these habits is not easy, but I know it's possible because many of my patients have done so. For some, it took a wake-up call—a heart attack, a diagnosis of cancer, or an emergency trip to the OR—to bring a change. Don't wait for such an event. Get the help you need to quit these addictions now. It could be the single best thing you do for your health and longevity.

A WORD ABOUT VAPING

In the past decade, vaping has become a mainstream habit for millions of Americans, especially teenagers and young adults. It involves inhaling an aerosol (a gaseous suspension of fine particles) that exposes your lungs to a variety of possibly toxic and carcinogenic chemicals.

Since vaping is a relatively recent phenomenon, there are no long-term studies on its health risks, but there have been numerous case reports of lung damage and deaths related to this activity. More research is required on its health consequences. Presently, it should not be considered a safe habit.

THINGS TO KNOW FOR HEALTH AND LONGEVITY

40. Good habits can enhance your health and longevity, while bad habits can undermine them.
41. There exists a real possibility of injury, illness, or even death from risk-taking behavior.
42. Be aware of the extensive damage from smoking— it's not just your lungs.
43. Be aware of the extensive damage from drinking— it's not just your liver.
44. Smoking and drinking can land you on an operating room table.
45. Stopping either smoking or drinking can be the single best thing you do for your health and longevity. If necessary, get professional help to quit.
46. Presently, vaping should not be considered a safe habit.

PART 2

NON-LIFESTYLE PRACTICES AND INTERVENTIONS FOR LONGEVITY

CHAPTER 5

HEALTH CONCEPTS FOR DETECTING AND PREVENTING DISEASES

"Bill, wake up. Dad needs your help. He's sick."

I remember the distress in my mom's voice when she said those words one early April morning in my house. I rushed downstairs to their bedroom and found my ninety-three-year-old father lethargic, barely able to speak, and unable to move his arms and legs. I thought he was having a massive stroke.

At the hospital, Eddie was found to be severely hyponatremic (he had low blood sodium). Due to this dangerous electrolyte abnormality, serious brain swelling occurred and caused his neurological condition. The damage was severe. My father would be bedridden for the next year, but miraculously he recovered almost completely from this episode. Sadly, it could have all been prevented.

A HEALTHY LIFESTYLE IS NOT ENOUGH

Eddie's lifestyle was responsible for much of his longevity, but I am sure that he wouldn't have made it to 101 on lifestyle alone. Even in someone with the healthiest lifestyle, illnesses will inevitably occur. What is important is that these afflictions are diagnosed early and treated appropriately.

Let's take, for example, Eddie's hypertension, which he developed at the age of eighty-two. Hypertension is a silent killer and was detected because the family routinely checked his blood pressure. With medication, this condition was well managed for the rest of his life. If it hadn't been discovered and treated, it could have caused serious harm to his body.

Non-lifestyle actions, such as screening for and managing hypertension, can play an important role in keeping you safe and healthy. Measures like this require that you learn and apply additional knowledge and skills. They involve the use of simple medical concepts, techniques, and equipment that could prevent diseases and injuries, as well as alert you to hidden conditions. They can even help you understand how to make better healthcare decisions.

SIGNS AND SYMPTOMS ARE IMPORTANT MESSAGES

Signs and symptoms play a valuable role in keeping you healthy. They are the clinical manifestations of a change from your usual state of well-being. They frequently indicate the presence of a pathological condition and are important clues the body provides to alert you that something is wrong.

Before we proceed further, let's clarify the technical difference between a sign and a symptom. Signs are objective evidence of an illness that can be seen or measured by others. A bruised arm, a swollen face, and a rapid heart rate are all signs. Symptoms are subjective and are what you experience. Weakness, dizziness, and pain are symptoms.

In everyday usage, the word "symptom" often refers to both a sign and a symptom. We frequently say the patient has the symptom of coughing, fever, or a lump. Coughing can be observed by others. A fever can be measured by others. And a lump can be seen or felt by others. Strictly speaking, they are all signs. But, for simplicity's sake, we will adopt the common understanding of the word "symptom" in this book.

Nonspecific Symptoms Are Easy to Ignore

Many symptoms are nonspecific. They don't point to an exact disease or body part or organ system. You have probably experienced the nonspecific symptom of fatigue when you had a cold, were overworked, or didn't sleep enough. But fatigue may also present itself in those with anemia, congestive heart failure, or chronic obstructive lung disease. A headache is another common symptom that is nonspecific. Its causes are diverse, including something as simple as missing your morning coffee—which deprives your body of caffeine—to serious etiologies, such as brain infections, bleeding, or tumors. One of the dangers of having a nonspecific symptom is that you may assign a harmless reason to it.

Be Aware of Diseases without Early Symptoms

Some diseases don't have any symptoms in their earlier stages. These diseases are insidious. They damage your health and endanger your life without you being aware of them until the they are in their late stages. Hypertension is a common example of an insidious disease—hence the nickname of "silent killer."

When Eddie was diagnosed with hypertension, he had never had any symptoms from the condition. He felt perfectly fine. Left undetected, this elevated blood pressure could have damaged his heart, brain, and kidneys without a trace of any pain or discomfort. It was only because we monitored his blood pressure regularly at home that this illness was detected.

Cancer is another insidious disease. It is the second leading cause of death in Americans. We fear it because it can strike unexpectedly. Symptoms may not appear until the cancer has grown into adjacent tissues and organs or has spread to other parts of the body. That is why preventive cancer screening tests, such as colonoscopies and mammograms, are so important. You must be vigilant about the symptoms of this disease.

Cancers can initially present as the following:
- Abnormal bleeding—blood in stool, blood in urine, postmenopausal or abnormal vaginal bleeding
- Changes in bowel habits—frequent bowel movements, persistent diarrhea or constipation, pencil-shaped stool
- Changes in urinary habits—difficulty urinating, painful urination, urinary frequency
- Changes in eating habits—difficulty swallowing foods, constant bloating after eating
- Lumps—a lump in the breast or on the testicle, persistent unexplained lumps anywhere in or on the body
- Skin changes—moles that are asymmetrical, irregularly shaped, and changing in size, color, or shape; sores that won't heal

- Chest symptoms—persistent cough, coughing up blood, recurrent lung infections
- Generalized symptoms—unexplained weight loss, fatigue, fever

All of these symptoms may or may not be cancer, but they should prompt you to seek medical attention.

Be Descriptive When Discussing Your Symptoms

Doctors collect information on your symptoms to arrive at a differential diagnosis. This is essentially a list of all the possible illnesses that you may have. You can help by providing a descriptive explanation that will guide them in their search for a diagnosis. Be honest, and don't be embarrassed to talk about any of your symptoms. An accurate and complete discussion is essential.

One of the most common symptoms is pain. Let's use it as an example of how you can describe a symptom to your doctor so they may start to uncover the condition that prompted you to seek medical attention.

Here are details of what you can tell your doctor about your pain:
- Location—Where is the pain? Does the pain move or radiate to other parts of the body?
- Timing—When did the pain start? Is it constant? When is it worse? When is it better?

- Description—Is the pain sharp, dull, aching, throbbing, cramping, or burning, or does it have other descriptive attributes?
- Intensity—How severe is the pain? On a scale of zero to ten, zero being no pain and ten being the worst pain imaginable, what number is it?
- Alleviating and exacerbating factors—What lessens the pain? What makes the pain worse?
- History—Is this pain new? Have you ever experienced this type of pain before?
- Associated symptoms—Is the pain associated with nausea, fever, chills, or any other symptoms?
- Effect on your life—Does the pain interfere with your ability to move about? To work? To sleep?

Many of the considerations that are applicable to pain are also relevant to other symptoms. It is good to be a prepared patient. You should think through and write down the pertinent points so that you don't forget them when you talk to your doctors.

Here are a few examples of how to describe your symptoms:

- "I have this constant stabbing pain at the base of my right big toe. It also feels stiff and hot. I don't remember hurting my toe. It just started by itself a couple of days ago, and it's getting worse. I can't even stand up now because it hurts so much."
- "I'm having severe sharp pain here (patient points to the upper-right portion of their abdomen) and I'm also feeling nauseous. I have a fever too. It all started yesterday after I ate dinner. I've had this type of pain

before, but it would only last an hour or so. This time, it won't go away."

- "I was feeling perfectly fine yesterday, but I woke up today with this dizziness and ringing in my ears. It's worse when I move my head. It feels like the room is spinning and I can't even walk straight."

Your doctors can make a list of likely diagnoses with just these brief but telling descriptions. You can play a more active role in your medical care by contributing essential information about your symptoms.

Persistent Symptoms Should Be Investigated

You can easily recognize the danger to your health when you experience symptoms such as crushing chest pain, labored breathing, or the sudden paralysis of an arm or leg. You know you must seek medical attention immediately. But other symptoms can appear harmless, in which case you may decide to treat them yourself—the persistent cough that just won't get better that you medicate with over-the-counter cough medicine, the chronic vague abdominal discomfort associated with bloating for which you take antacids, and the daily morning headaches that you try to alleviate with an assortment of pain relievers. These symptoms are nonspecific and can be caused by benign conditions, but the same symptoms can also be warning signs of something more serious.

Eddie once had symptoms that I managed instead of having the real problem diagnosed and treated. It resulted in his life-threatening encounter with hyponatremia. It was a mistake that could have been avoided.

On my dad's ninety-third birthday, he could still walk briskly and climb stairs without difficulty. Half a year later, I noticed a change. His steps became slow and deliberate. He started to lean backward as he walked, as if he was compensating for an imbalance in his body. He even slipped and fell a couple of times when attempting to stand up from a chair. He would laugh about it and say, "This old car is falling apart."

The changes occurred gradually, over a span of a couple of months. He had no other complaints during this time, so I (and he) thought his weakness and the changes in his gait and balance were simply due to his body aging—after all, my dad was in his nineties. I treated his symptoms by buying him a cane and a walker to use instead of getting him a medical workup. A simple blood test would have uncovered his hyponatremia. The progression of this abnormality could have been stopped, and that catastrophic neurological event on that early April morning could have been prevented. Not getting a workup is something I've always regretted.

Don't manage persistent symptoms—even the ones that appear harmless—by yourself. They should be medically evaluated to rule out the possibility of a serious hidden condition.

PREVENTIVE HEALTHCARE IS A MUST

When it came to seeking healthcare, Eddie was old-school. If he didn't feel sick, he thought nothing could be wrong and there was no need to see a doctor. He only sought medical help when he absolutely had to. So it took quite a bit of coercion to finally convince him to go for routine annual checkups. I told him that it was like taking a car for its yearly inspection to make sure it was still safe to drive—like a car, there could be hidden problems. This analogy he understood.

Preventive healthcare is essential, even if you feel well and think you are in good health. Since many diseases can be insidious, they can only be found if your doctors actively look for them. As you age, it is even more crucial to pursue preventive care because your risks of many illnesses increase significantly.

The importance of detecting a medical condition early cannot be overstated. Early discovery allows for more treatment options, better management of the disease, and possibly a cure. This is especially true for some cancers, for which there are routine screening exams that can detect malignancies in their initial and precancerous stages. When performed in a timely fashion, these exams may even prevent the development of the disease.

In the operating room, I have cared for many patients who could have avoided major surgeries and given themselves a better chance for survival if they had found their cancer in its initial stages or before it metastasized. You must take advantage of available cancer screening exams as part of your preventive healthcare routine. Consult your healthcare provider to determine at what age and how often you should be screened and which tests are best for you. Don't just wait until symptoms appear.

At present, here are some available cancer screening exams:

COLORECTAL

- Colonoscopy—direct visualization technique, which is the most invasive of the colorectal screening exams but has the advantage of being the most thorough; polyps (fleshy growths that start off as benign but may become cancerous) can be detected and the majority of them removed at the time of the procedure

- Sigmoidoscopy—direct visualization exam of only the rectum and sigmoid parts of the colon, where most of the colorectal cancers occur
- Computed tomography (CT) colonography or virtual colonoscopy—radiological study of the colon
- Fecal tests—examination of stool for evidence of blood and DNA markers of colorectal cancers

BREAST

- Self-examination—monthly breast self-exams should start by the age of twenty; they are especially important for those women younger than their recommended age for a mammogram; self-exams should be performed between your screening mammograms and should never replace your mammograms
- Mammogram—primary screening tool for breast cancer in the United States; can detect abnormal breast tissue too small to be felt by physical exam
- Ultrasound—may be recommended along with mammogram for patients with dense breast tissue
- Genetic testing—laboratory analysis of blood or saliva for gene mutations may be recommended in patients with a strong family history of breast cancer

CERVICAL

- Pap test—looks for precancerous changes in cells from the cervix

- HPV test—detects the presence of HPV (human papillomavirus) infection, which is the main risk factor for cervical cancer

PROSTATE

- PSA test—blood test for PSA (prostate-specific antigen); note that controversy exists as to the use of PSA screening due to the risks of overdiagnosing and overtreating prostate cancers, some of which are slow growing and may not cause any health problems during the patient's lifetime

LUNG

- Low-dose CT scan of the lungs—may be recommended for smokers based on age, as well as on how much and for how many years they smoked

A SIMPLE MEASURE TO REDUCE THE RISK OF LUNG CANCER

In the United States, lung cancer kills more people than any other cancer. Yearly deaths from lung cancer exceed those from colon, breast, and cervical cancers combined. Cigarette smoking is the leading cause of lung cancer and radon is the second. It is estimated that approximately twenty thousand Americans will die from radon-related cancers of the lungs each year.

Radon is a carcinogen. Invisible and odorless, it's a radioactive gas that comes from the breakdown of uranium that is naturally found in soil. It can enter and collect in your home through foundation cracks and openings, exposing you and your family to potentially high levels of this carcinogen. Radon can also enter through well water. It is estimated that almost one out of every fifteen homes in the United States has an elevated level. The only way to know how much radon is in your house is to screen for it. Inexpensive and easy-to-use kits are available for this purpose. They may be readily purchased at major hardware stores or online.

I know personally about radon. A few years after my family moved into our house, I purchased a kit and, to my surprise, the results showed significantly elevated levels of this gas in my home. I really didn't expect the level to be high, since I live in a low-radon area, according to the United States Environmental Protection Agency Map of Radon Zones. (Note that the EPA recommends testing for all homes, regardless of the zone.) I repeated the test with additional kits, which confirmed the high readings. This prompted me to immediately seek remediation with a qualified radon professional. A mitigation system of fans, pipes, and vents was subsequently installed to suction out the cancer-causing gas from below the house and release it into the air outside. This resolved the problem, and the radon in my home is now at a low, safe level.

Screening for radon was an important preventive step I took to protect my family's health. You should do the same. You don't know if you are exposing yourself and your loved ones to dangerous amounts of this carcinogen unless you test for it.

VACCINATIONS PROTECT YOU FROM INFECTIOUS DISEASES

After he started his annual checkups, Eddie always kept up to date with his flu and pneumonia vaccinations. I believe the vaccines, in combination with our infection preventive measures at home, helped protect my father from catching any contagious respiratory ailments in the latter years of his life.

Keeping up your vaccinations is important. With the advent of the recent pandemic, the public has again recognized the vital role that vaccines play in our health. Routine vaccinations are an effective measure to reduce the risks of contracting infectious diseases, such as the common flu, pneumococcal pneumonia, and COVID-19. This is especially critical for the elderly population and those with serious pre-existing conditions, who are at a greater risk of severe infection and death from these illnesses.

PROTECT YOUR BODY'S COMPLEX CHEMISTRY

Think of the body as a chemical reactor where trillions of chemical reactions are occurring every second to keep you alive. These reactions vary, from the processes that release energy from the foods you eat to the processes that create the necessary proteins for life, such as hormones and enzymes. These reactions preserve homeostasis—the maintenance of a stable internal body environment that involves regulating body temperature, blood pressure, and blood sugar levels, among other vital functions. And let's not forget, they make you who you are—they somehow create your consciousness, memories, and the emotions that you experience.

These chemical activities taking place in your body are remarkably complex. Take, for example, the reactions that occur to produce sleep when anesthetic drugs are given. Although anesthetics have been utilized for over a century and a half, and hundreds of millions of patients are safely anesthetized throughout the world every year, anesthesiologists still don't know how anesthesia works. They don't understand the exact cellular mechanisms of the drugs they administer, despite all the science that exists today to research this mystery. They can't explain on a molecular level how these medications transition a patient's state of consciousness into one of unconsciousness. It's a mystery because the human body's chemistry is so complex.

It is important to recognize this complexity so you are aware that whatever you expose yourself to—whatever you let into your reactor—can interact with your unique and intricate chemistry. This includes molecules of drugs, supplements, pollutants, and other chemicals. Exposure to any of these could result in physiological changes, many of which cannot be predicted and some of which will be harmful.

All Drugs Can Cause Adverse Reactions

Pharmaceutical drugs are molecules specifically designed to interact beneficially with your body's chemistry. They can cure or help manage many diseases, improve your quality of life, and increase longevity. Eddie's antihypertensive medicine lowered his blood pressure to normal levels, decreasing his chances of cardiovascular complications. But along with their benefits, all medications are associated with possible adverse reactions.

It is impossible to predict all the potential outcomes that can occur with newly discovered pharmaceuticals, due to the complexity of the body's chemistry. For this reason, in order for a new drug to receive Food and Drug Administration (FDA) approval, it must go through an extensive series of trials. Multiple studies of sufficient size and scope are required to answer the following questions: Will the novel drug work? What side effects will appear? Do the benefits outweigh the risks?

Unwanted reactions to medication can be allergy-related or can be side effects of the drug. Allergic symptoms appear due to an abnormal immune response to the chemical composition of the medicine. One of the most common drug allergies that doctors encounter is penicillin. The reaction to penicillin can range from a mild skin rash and hives to full blown, life-threatening anaphylaxis.

Side effects are much more common than allergic reactions. At times, they are unpredictable and may be related to an individual's unique chemical makeup. Most of the adverse effects are minor, such as an upset stomach or a dry mouth, but serious consequences can arise, as with Eddie's hyponatremia.

Dietary Supplements Are Not Always Harmless

Drugs are only one of a number of agents that can interact with your body's chemistry. Many Americans take dietary supplements—vitamins, minerals, amino acids, enzymes, and herbs, for example—believing that they are harmless, but they, too, can have bad health effects.

Supplements have been linked to elevated cancer risks, increased bleeding, and toxicity to organs such as the liver. Because they are not categorized as drugs by the FDA, they do not have to pass the same rigorous testing that drugs do. Be especially careful about taking megadose supplements unless they are prescribed or recommended by your physician. You must recognize that risks exist with these bioactive agents.

Non-pharmaceutical Chemicals Can Cause Serious Health Consequences

Chemicals are everywhere. They are in the air we breathe, the food we eat, and the products we touch. They have enriched our lives in many ways, making our drinking water clean, increasing our agricultural food production, and providing energy and materials for the world we live in. However, some chemicals are harmful, and your body's exposure to these agents can result in potentially serious health consequences.

Reactions to chemicals can vary from toxic (lead poisoning) to carcinogenic (cancer from cigarette smoke) to allergic (latex sensitivities). The effect can be immediate, such as the sudden onset of headaches and dizziness from inhaling solvent fumes, or arise decades later, with the development of lung cancer after exposure to asbestos.

Chemicals can't harm you unless they get into your body. You can inhale them when you breathe in second-hand smoke or soot from a wood-burning fireplace. You can consume them when you eat pesticides left on fruits and vegetables or when you drink water contaminated with arsenic and nitrates. You can even absorb them through your skin. Dermal exposure to potentially harmful agents, such as solvents (acetone, formaldehyde, and benzene found in some beauty products), can produce measurable levels of these substances in the blood.

So how do you protect yourself? The most important action you can take is to be aware and careful of what you let into your body.

Here are some simple things you can do to protect your body's complex chemistry from harmful reactions:
- Take only necessary medications and health supplements.
- Wash fruits and vegetables thoroughly to remove dirt and pesticides.

- Microwave food in glass or Pyrex cookware and not in plastic food containers (when microwaved, some plastics release bisphenol-A and phthalates, which are chemicals that disrupt your body's hormonal system).
- Be aware of what is in your cleaning and personal care products.
- Avoid breathing in chemicals, exhaust fumes, and particulate matter (powders, dust, smoke, soot) by staying a safe distance away, ventilating the area, or wearing an appropriate protective mask.
- Handle chemicals with care by wearing appropriate protective gloves and eyewear.

MAKE BETTER HEALTHCARE DECISIONS

At the age of eighty-eight, Eddie had an acute episode of upper abdominal pain. After appropriate medical evaluations, no specific cause of the symptom was found, although a mass was incidentally discovered in his gallbladder on one of his radiological tests. This lesion could have been benign or malignant, but if it was cancerous or would become a cancer, the prognosis would be poor. A decision had to be made: surgically remove the gallbladder or follow this growth over time with various scanning exams, hoping there would be no change in the lesion. The family had to weigh the benefits and risks of each of the treatment plans. We had to apply what I call **BRAT** analysis.

Benefits, Risks, and Alternative Treatments (**BRAT**) can help you understand and evaluate therapeutic options.

When your doctor prescribes a new medication, orders a test, or recommends a procedure, think and apply **BRAT**. What are the benefits? What are the risks? Do the benefits outweigh the risks? Are there any alternative treatments or tests? Having your doctor answer these questions will provide you with valuable knowledge and insights that will help you make better healthcare choices. It will also increase your awareness of possible side effects and complications if you decide to proceed.

How to Weigh Benefits versus Risks

Weighing benefits versus risks seems intuitive—like comparing a list of pros and cons—but there is more to it. In addition to weighing the value of the benefits and the severity of the risks, you must also consider the likelihood of either good or bad outcomes occurring before you determine if it is prudent to proceed. For example, the most serious of risks—death—is usually not acceptable unless the probability of dying is very low. Whether you recognize it or not, you accept this risk when you drive a car, fly in an airplane, or consent to having anesthesia.

When assessing benefit versus risk, the factors you need to consider can be charted to help you think through your options.

The best scenario would be an option that offers the combination of maximum benefits and a high likelihood of them occurring, together with harmless risks that most likely will not even appear. The worst scenario would be an intervention with minimal benefits and a small chance of them occurring, associated with a high probability of severe risks. Almost all situations will fall between these two extremes.

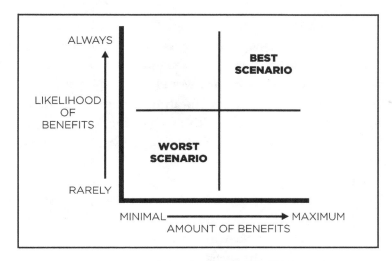

CHARTING BENEFITS

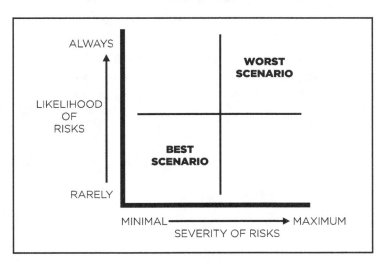

CHARTING RISKS

Applying BRAT to Eddie's Case

For my father's gallbladder lesion, there was the option of surgery or the alternative treatment of watching and waiting. Each choice had its own set of risks and benefits. An operation would remove the cancer or the chance of cancer developing from the mass—maximum benefits with high probability. The main hazard would be complications from the surgery or the anesthetic in an elderly patient—mild to moderate severity of risks with low likelihood of complications (largely in part because of Eddie's overall good health and fitness).

If, instead, the family decided to watch and wait, the obvious benefit would be no harm to Eddie from the procedure or the anesthetic. But with waiting, there exists the real possibility of gallbladder cancer with its bad prognosis. In the end, my father opted for the operation, and he did well.

Making healthcare decisions can be extremely difficult and stressful. At times, there may not be a right or wrong choice that applies to everyone, because how each of us views the benefits and risks is different. What is always needed, however, is a thorough discussion of **BRAT** with your doctors so that you can make the best possible informed decision.

THINGS TO KNOW FOR HEALTH AND LONGEVITY

47. Non-lifestyle measures are essential for good health and longevity.

48. Symptoms are important warning signals.

49. Many diseases are insidious and therefore more dangerous.

50. Be alert to the early signs of cancer.

51. A detailed description of symptoms can help your doctor make the proper diagnosis.

52. Persistent symptoms should be evaluated; don't ignore them or just treat them yourself.

53. Preventive healthcare is essential, even if you feel well or think you are healthy.

54. Always get your cancer screening exams.

55. Test your home for radon.

56. Keep up with your vaccinations.

57. Your body is a collection of complex chemical reactions.

58. Be aware of what drugs, supplements, and chemicals you expose your body to.

59. All medications, medical tests, and procedures have benefits and risks.

60. Use **BRAT** when you talk with your healthcare providers.

61. Use **BRAT** to make better healthcare decisions.

CHAPTER 6

LIFESAVING PHYSIOLOGICAL MONITORING AT HOME

The prognosis was grave. A few days after his hyponatremic event, Eddie still was unable to move his arms and his legs. He was more alert, but he could barely speak and could not eat solid foods.

The medical consultants estimated that it would be a few weeks, at most, before he succumbed to his illness. I was well aware of my dad's wishes to be at home during the last days of his life, so I spoke to his attending physician about discharging him to my house for hospice care. The doctor agreed to the early discharge—at least he would be with family and in familiar surroundings when he passed away.

So just three days after his admission to the hospital, Eddie was sent home directly from the intensive care unit. Before he arrived, we made the necessary arrangements. A hospital bed was delivered, as well as an oxygenator, a machine that concentrated oxygen from the air for my dad to breathe.

*To medically monitor him, I had a blood pressure
machine, an electrocardiogram (ECG) monitor, and a
pulse oximeter. With these devices—along with lots of
love, work, and care from his wife and family—Eddie
made a remarkable recovery and lived for another eight
good years.*

PHYSIOLOGICAL MONITORING GIVES US VITAL INFORMATION

During anesthesia, physiological monitoring is essential—your operating room experience is much safer because of it. Administering anesthesia without using any monitoring devices or techniques is like driving without headlights during a moonless night, in total darkness: you don't know where you are, and you don't know when or which way to turn. Anesthesiologists must have information on what is physiologically happening to your body to carry you safely through an operation.

At home, the monitors I placed in Eddie's room guided me in managing his recovery. I used an ECG to make sure his heart rate was regular and wasn't too fast or too slow. Abnormal heart rhythms and rates can provide clues to underlying disease processes. Since Eddie had a history of hypertension, I followed his blood pressure closely with an automatic machine to confirm that it was still under control. More importantly, I looked for hypotension (low blood pressure) to alert me to possible dehydration as well as other conditions related to his cardiovascular system. I additionally took advantage of a pulse oximeter, an amazing device. It provided me with essential information on how well oxygen was being delivered from his lungs to his blood. Its readings helped to determine the amount of nasal cannula oxygen I should provide and how aggressive we needed to be with pulmonary maneuvers. These actions included repositioning his body to breathe better, percussing or striking his back with cupped hands to loosen the secretions in his lungs, and getting him to cough and take deeper inhalations and exhalations in an attempt to open up his respiratory airways.

These efforts, along with numerous other interventions— intravenous fluids when he appeared dehydrated, antibiotics when he developed signs of infection, and egg drop soup that he sipped for months when he was unable to eat solid food— led to his unbelievable recovery.

WHAT CAN HOME PHYSIOLOGICAL MONITORING DO FOR YOU?

Physiological monitoring was critical to the management of Eddie's illness. Without the information it provided, he wouldn't have survived. It saved his life, and it can also be used in your home to possibly save your life or the life of a loved one.

Most people overlook self-monitoring and the role it can play in their health. To many people, physiological monitoring belongs in a doctor's office or a hospital and there's no reason to familiarize oneself with it. But it's a tool that is valuable and available, and it should be taken advantage of to maximize your chances of living a long life.

Now I'm not referring to employing monitors in the same capacity as they were used to direct Eddie's care. Self-monitoring is not about applying advanced modalities that only medical personnel can perform and comprehend. Instead, what you will learn are a few simple ways to use monitoring devices and techniques to help you stay healthy and to alert you to conditions that require medical attention.

YOUR LONGEVITY DEPENDS ON OXYGEN

Let's talk a bit here about oxygen and its essential role for life, because it's ultimately the reason why doctors use monitoring equipment. This is something you need to appreciate if you truly want to understand the basis for your health and longevity. How healthy you stay and how long you live will depend on how well your body continues to deliver precious oxygen molecules to its cells.

You have a heart attack because your heart muscle isn't getting enough oxygen. You have a stroke when a part of your brain is deprived of oxygen. And you bleed to death due to the loss of the body's ability to deliver oxygen. Throughout the COVID-19 crisis, doctors were constantly concerned about patients' oxygen numbers—and for good reason. Low oxygenation levels indicated and led to more serious disease, as vital organs were deprived of this essential element.

Although it is not as evident, even the main danger of Eddie's hyponatremia came from a problem with oxygen. With his low blood sodium level, severe brain swelling occurred. This expansion of tissue within the fixed volume of his skull increased his intracranial pressure, which, in turn, led to a serious reduction in blood flow to parts of his brain. Inadequate cerebral blood flow meant inadequate oxygen delivery and subsequent neuron dysfunction and death. So ultimately, it was the lack of oxygen in Eddie's brain cells that caused his neurological deterioration.

You can see that anything that decreases the transport of oxygen to your tissues is dangerous. But precisely why is this so? What is it about oxygen that makes it so important?

Simply put, oxygen makes possible the energy for living. Through a series of intracellular chemical reactions called cellular respiration, oxygen is used to make adenosine triphosphate (ATP), the molecule that provides energy for your tissues and organs. ATP is utilized ubiquitously throughout your body, from muscle contractions to DNA synthesis to intracellular functions. Without ATP, your cells cannot survive. Unfortunately, your body cannot store much ATP; it must be produced continuously.

Your brain is the organ that is the most sensitive to the deprivation of oxygen. It takes only five minutes without oxygen to deplete your brain's ATP energy reserves. With no energy for your neurons to maintain their life-sustaining processes, brain death quickly ensues. That is why it's so vital to sustain well-oxygenated blood flow, so that this process of energy production is kept intact.

FEEL A PULSE TO SAVE A LIFE

In the operating room, one of the primary reasons we use an electrocardiogram monitor is to detect arrhythmias. At home, instead of an ECG, you can learn to monitor for an irregular heart rhythm by applying the simple technique of palpating a pulse. Twice in my life, outside of a medical setting, I detected life-threatening arrhythmias by simply feeling someone's radial pulse and sensing its rhythm. Sure, it helped that I am an anesthesiologist, but believe me, you can do it too. It just takes practice.

Eddie never had any problems with arrhythmias, but Wai, my mother, did. One morning, I saw her in the kitchen making breakfast. She appeared to be her usual healthy and active eighty-six-year-old self but mentioned to me that she was a bit lightheaded. She wasn't dizzy, didn't feel like fainting, and didn't have any trouble going about her day. She simply noticed there was something different in the way she was feeling. It was hard for Wai to describe her symptoms.

Her complaints were vague and didn't appear serious. But just to be sure, I reached out, put my fingers on my mother's wrist, and felt for the radial pulse. It was such an easy maneuver that provided critical information about her condition. In less than a minute, I discovered that the rhythm of her pulse was very irregular. The beats of her pulse occurred randomly—I felt some immediately after another, some after a short pause, and some after a long pause. There was no predictability as to when I would feel the next beat.

This finding was new for Wai. She didn't have a prior history of an irregular heart rhythm, so I knew right then that this was a medical emergency. Within a couple of hours, she was seen by a cardiologist, who confirmed the diagnosis of atrial fibrillation (AFib) and immediately started on anticoagulant medication to prevent a stroke, one of the most dangerous complications of this arrhythmia.

The other time I uncovered an irregular heart rhythm outside of work was with another senior family member. He was at a family birthday party when he felt very tired—so much so that he had to lie down. When I went to check on him, he complained only of feeling weak. I felt his pulse and, again, within a minute, I recognized that this, too, was a medical emergency. He needed to go immediately to the hospital.

In minutes, we were in the car and on our way. In the emergency room, the electrocardiogram monitor showed AFib with occasional outbreaks of sustained ventricular tachycardia, an even more serious life-threatening arrhythmia. He was treated with intravenous antiarrhythmics and blood thinning drugs, and admitted to the coronary care unit.

It's important to realize that, in both these cases, neither my mother nor my other relative had any severe complaints. They would not have sought medical care if I hadn't bothered to feel their pulse—a simple, convenient, and quick monitoring technique. Left undiscovered, the irregular heart rhythms could have led to a stroke or a sudden cardiac event, including cardiac arrest and death.

How to Feel for the Radial Pulse and Sense Its Rhythm

A pulse is a palpable wave of blood that is generated by the contraction of the heart. This pulse wave travels throughout the arteries of the body and can be best felt at the wrist, neck, and groin. Each pulse you detect represents a heartbeat. The number of pulses you feel per minute normally corresponds to your heart rate.

The pulse of the radial artery can be felt on the thumb side of your wrist. Using a moderate amount of pressure, place your index and middle fingers along the wrist creases, below your thumb. You may sense the pulse right away. If you don't, slowly slide your fingertips sideways, in tiny increments, along the creases. You may notice two prominent cord-like structures (tendons) in the middle of your wrist. Always stay to the thumb side of these tendons. Vary your finger pressure to learn what amount of force is best for your digits to detect the wave of blood. If you practice enough, it should take only a minute or less (usually seconds) to find the radial pulse in most individuals.

When you feel the pulse, note its rhythm. It may be fast or slow, but it should be regular and steady. You can tap out or sound out the beats of the pulse and predict when the next beat will occur. Try it. You can have an occasional extra or skipped beat, but overall the beats should be occurring regularly. With an irregular rhythm, there is no predictability or pattern to the pulse. The beats seem to occur haphazardly. If you detect an irregular pulse, seek medical attention.

There are now smart devices, including smartwatches, that can produce a simplified electrocardiogram reading to help detect AFib and other abnormal heart rhythms. They should be considered a potentially important part of your physiological monitoring tools.

FOLLOW YOUR BLOOD PRESSURE TO DETECT HYPERTENSION, A SILENT KILLER

When Eddie turned eighty-one years old, he still didn't have any chronic health conditions—no heart disease, no lung disease, and no diabetes or hypertension. At that point in his life, I was already checking his blood pressure regularly (every month or so), and it always stayed in the lower range of normal. Then, over the course of a single year, I watched as his numbers began to slowly increase and then accelerate upward until the values qualified my father for a diagnosis of hypertension. Throughout this period, Eddie had no symptoms. Without the home monitoring, this elevation in his blood pressure would have gone undetected.

Hypertension is the single most significant risk factor for heart disease and stroke. It is also one of the most common reasons for kidney failure. Yet elevated blood pressures causes few or no symptoms until significant damage has been done to the body's organ systems. That is why it is important to monitor your blood pressure routinely—to help yourself and your doctor detect and manage this silent killer.

Understanding Blood Pressure Numbers

Blood pressure is expressed as two numbers—for example, 110/70, which is read as 110 over 70. The first, or upper, number is your systolic reading. It's the pressure in your arteries in millimeters of mercury (mm Hg) that is generated by your heart during its contraction. The second, or lower, number is your diastolic reading. It's the pressure in your arteries between the contractions, when the heart's main pumping chamber is at rest.

Both numbers are important to your health. An elevation of either the systolic or diastolic number can be considered hypertension. In 2017, the American College of Cardiology (ACC) / American Heart Association (AHA) Task Force released its new *Guideline for the Prevention, Detection, Evaluation and Management of High Blood Pressure in Adults.*

THE HYPERTENSION CATEGORIES FROM THE ACC/AHA GUIDELINES			
BLOOD PRESSURE CATEGORY	SYSTOLIC NUMBER	AND/ OR	DIASTOLIC NUMBER
Normal	less than 120	and	less than 80
Elevated	120 to 129	and	less than 80
Hypertension Stage 1	130 to 139	or	80 to 89
Hypertension Stage 2	140 or higher	or	90 or higher

For the first time in over a decade, the task force redefined the numbers for hypertension. Previously, the AHA defined hypertension as 140/90 and higher; the new definition is 130 and higher for the systolic number *or* 80 and higher for the diastolic reading. This more generous definition of hypertension was adopted to promote earlier intervention of this damaging disease process.

Following the updated guideline, a normal blood pressure is now less than 120/80. It is estimated that, with the new numbers, close to half of the American adult population is now classified as having "elevated" or hypertensive blood pressure. This makes home blood pressure monitoring even more valuable.

How Does Hypertension Damage Your Body?

Eddie thought of his heart as an engine. He believed this muscular organ provided the energy for his muscles to move via the blood that it pushed throughout the body. It was just like a combustible engine that produces the energy to drive a car, he speculated.

His analogy was not quite right. The reality is that the blood itself does not carry energy; it carries fuel (oxygen) to the muscle cells so that they can create energy (ATP) locally to power the movements of the body.

It is more accurate to think of the heart as a pump and the arteries as tubing connected to it. In this simplistic model, imagine the pump pushing a fluid through the tubing. If the lumen (inside space of a tubular structure) of the tubing is narrowed, as with the arteries in a hypertensive person, the pressure that is required to move a given amount of fluid in a set amount of time is increased. With higher pressure, the flow of fluid causes more shear stress on the tubing and can damage the tubing—or, in the case of a human body, can damage the cells that make up the inner lining of the arteries.

The constant higher pressure in the system will also increase the workload and wear and tear on the pump, damaging it. The same will happen to your heart. Any appliance (organ) connected to the tubing that is exposed to an increased pressure load will also suffer. In terms of your body, your brain, kidneys, and even the retinas of your eyes will be subjected to the detrimental effects of the elevated pressures, resulting in injury to these structures. All this damage inflicted by hypertension eventually translates into a higher risk of heart and cerebrovascular disease, dementia, and renal failure.

Chronic hypertensive disease is dangerous, but acute, severe upward spikes in blood pressure can be especially hazardous to your immediate health. These spikes may be triggered by emotions such as fear and anger. These extreme pressures can create excessive strain on the heart, leading to pump or cardiac failure. The increased workload on this organ will also elevate its oxygen demands and, if an insufficient amount of oxygen is delivered to the cardiac muscles, a heart attack can ensue. Moreover, just as a piece of tubing or a pipe can leak or burst due to high pressure, the blood vessels in the brain can rupture from severe hypertension, resulting in a stroke. Studies have shown that, after an episode of anger, your chance of a stroke triples. There is a reason why people say, "control your temper or you'll have a stroke."

Measuring Your Blood Pressure Correctly

There are two major reasons to monitor your blood pressure at home. One is to detect hypertension that is not picked up in your doctor's office. A single blood pressure number obtained during a routine checkup is just an isolated snapshot of a continuum of possible readings. Regular home measurements can identify a blood pressure problem that is missed in medical settings. If you already have a history of hypertension, the second reason to self-monitor is to document how your blood pressure is responding to medications or lifestyle changes.

Here are a few important pointers on blood pressure monitoring:

- Buy an automatic blood pressure device. It is easier to use, especially when checking your own numbers.
- Make sure you have the correct-size cuff. The wrong size can result in an unreliable reading. Too small a cuff may result in higher blood pressure numbers and too large a cuff in lower numbers.
- Place your upper arm at approximately the level of your heart. The position of your upper arm can affect the measurement. If you place it above the heart, the value may be falsely lower. If you place it below the heart, the value may be falsely higher.
- Take your measurements at rest and not immediately after exercising or smoking. Wait at least half an hour after these activities.
- Take the reading two or three times, separated by a minute or two, just to ensure that the readings are consistent.
- Take a set of measurements twice a day—once in the morning and once in the evening.
- Bring your blood pressure machine to your doctor's office to check if your machine's readings match their readings. Do this test to evaluate the accuracy of your device.

A journal of recorded blood pressure measurements is helpful to your physician for the diagnosis and management of hypertension. How frequently you need to monitor your numbers will depend on your medical history. Ask your doctor for guidance.

A PULSE OXIMETER PROVIDES CRITICAL INFORMATION

The pulse oximeter is a remarkable piece of engineering ingenuity. It's painless, noninvasive, and easy to use. It provides critical information—your blood oxygen saturation. Just clip it onto your finger and a reading usually appears within seconds. Previously, a specimen of blood had to be taken from an artery and processed through a blood gas analyzer machine.

The ability to monitor blood oxygen saturation has prevented countless numbers of dangerous hypoxic (low body tissue oxygenation) events in the operating room, saving the lives of many patients. Without a doubt, it is one of the most important monitors in an anesthesiologist's toolbox. Before the routine use of this instrument, doctors had to look for changes in vital signs or cyanosis (the bluish or purplish discoloration of the skin or the lips) to alert them to inadequate blood oxygen levels.

When Eddie was bedridden, I was concerned about him developing many of the complications associated with a prolonged inability to move. High up on the list was an increased risk of pulmonary problems. Atelectasis (collapsed lung tissue), pneumonia, and other lung infections could have readily developed due to his constant recumbent position. Another concern was pulmonary embolism. His lack of movement elevated the risk of blood clots forming in his legs. Pieces of these clots could then have been released into the veins and circulated into the heart and out to the lungs, resulting in low blood oxygen levels. With the pulse oximeter, I monitored for decreasing oxygenation readings, which could indicate the presence of these conditions.

What the Pulse Oximeter Can Be Used For

Athletes have been taking advantage of pulse oximeters for years. Those who engage in high-altitude activities rely on the devices to help them assess their body's response to low-oxygen environments. Participants in endurance sports may use pulse oximeters to guide their training and recovery routines as well as their breathing techniques.

Doctors prescribe pulse oximeters for the monitoring of acute and chronic diseases that impair breathing. The information provided by a pulse oximeter can direct patients and their physicians on the use of home-based oxygen therapy, much as it did during Eddie's recovery. During the COVID-19 crisis, many people purchased one of these devices to detect low blood oxygen levels—to alert them to one of the signs of the infection or to follow the course of a documented infection.

One of the invaluable strengths of a pulse oximeter is that it can provide evidence of a hidden disease process. A low saturation number may be the first clue to an undiagnosed lung or heart condition. It gives you a warning that something is wrong and that you need to see a doctor.

Understanding What a Pulse Oximeter Measures

You must understand the pulse oximeter's reading in order to use the device wisely. This instrument measures oxygen saturation, but what exactly is that? You need to comprehend a bit of physiology to fully grasp what it is and why it's important.

Oxygen in your blood is carried by hemoglobin molecules in your red blood cells (RBCs). These molecules have multiple binding sites that can hold oxygen. If all the hemoglobin sites in your RBCs are completely occupied, the pulse oximeter will show a reading of 100 percent oxygen saturation. If an average of 80 percent of the sites are occupied, the reading will be 80 percent. The oximeter essentially measures the percentage of binding sites that are taken up by oxygen. The higher the oxygen saturation, the more oxygen is being carried in your blood for a given amount of hemoglobin.

A normal oxygen saturation is 95 to 100 percent, and a lower reading usually indicates a lung or heart condition. Be aware that a saturation of 90 percent or less is considered critical and warrants immediate medical attention. Just as important as the number itself is its trend. Oximeter measurements that are decreasing over time are of concern and also should be evaluated.

Oxygen Deficiency with a High Saturation Number

Can your body be deficient of oxygen with an oximeter reading of 100 percent? The answer is yes. But how is this possible?

An analogy can help us understand the answer to this question. Think of hemoglobin as a grocery bag and oxygen as the food you put into it. If the bag is totally filled with food—similar to hemoglobin sites completely occupied by oxygen—it can be considered 100 percent saturated. Say you need five of these 100 percent saturated bags of groceries for a party. If you have only one of these bags, clearly there will not be enough food for your guests to eat. Similarly, if there is a deficiency of hemoglobin (or red blood cells containing the hemoglobin), there will not be enough oxygen to meet your body's needs, regardless of a high oxygen saturation number.

You can also apply the exaggeration trick we discussed in Chapter 1 to further comprehend this scenario. Imagine you have just a single red blood cell in your body and its hemoglobin is fully bound with oxygen; the pulse oximeter will theoretically read 100 percent. Obviously, there is not enough oxygen for your organs and tissues.

Severe anemia can be one cause of oxygen deprivation in the setting of high oxygen saturation numbers, but there are other reasons too. Users of pulse oximeters should know that while low readings should be medically evaluated, normal or high values don't necessarily mean that things are clinically well. In other words, if you feel the need to seek medical help, don't let any pulse oximeter number stop you from doing so.

How to Use a Pulse Oximeter

Pulse oximeters are readily available and may be purchased from local pharmacies, big general retail stores, and online sites. A prescription is unnecessary for a device that is not FDA cleared. These over-the-counter oximeters do not undergo required FDA clinical testing to verify their accuracy. If you have an ailment that necessitates home oxygen saturation monitoring, consult with your doctor and have your doctor prescribe an FDA-approved device.

Here are a few important pointers on using a pulse oximeter:
- Any finger can be used for monitoring, as long as the pulse oximeter fits securely and produces a steady reading.

- Avoid shaking or moving your finger while using the device.
- Cold hands or any conditions that reduce circulation to your fingers can lead to difficulties in obtaining a measurement and can generate inaccurate numbers.
- Artificial fingernails may affect the ability of the oximeter to pick up a reading (you can use your toes instead).
- Carbon monoxide exposure from smoking or carbon monoxide poisoning can produce falsely elevated readings.

A NORMAL THERMOMETER READING DOES NOT RULE OUT INFECTIONS

You already know that a thermometer is a useful monitoring instrument to have at home. It detects or confirms the presence of a fever, which is commonly associated with an infectious process. I used it frequently during the time my dad was incapacitated.

While bedridden, Eddie had a significantly increased risk of developing an infection from three primary sources: his lungs, his Foley catheter (a tube placed in his bladder for urine drainage), and decubitus ulcers (pressure bedsores). As part of a daily search for this condition, I used a thermometer to check whether he was febrile. Besides measuring his temperature, I also looked for general symptoms, such as lethargy and loss of appetite, and more specific clues, such as abnormal lung sounds, cloudy urine, and redness around the bedsores, as evidence of an infectious process. Even without an elevated temperature, I would frequently start my dad on antibiotics if he had any of these signs.

As with all other monitoring devices, thermometers have limitations that must be recognized in order for you to use them safely. You should be aware that the absence of a fever doesn't rule out the presence of a bacterial or viral illness. Especially with the elderly, a normal body temperature can exist even in the face of a serious active infection. So don't let a normal thermometer reading prevent you from consulting your doctor if you suspect such a condition.

FITNESS TRACKERS PROVIDE OBJECTIVE DATA

You can monitor your pulse rhythm, blood pressure, and oxygen saturation to help you stay in good health—so why not monitor your activity level too? As you know, an adequate amount of physical activity is essential for staying healthy and living a long life. It was a key part of Eddie's longevity story.

A wearable device such as a fitness tracker can monitor and record the number of steps you take during the day or for a particular activity. It can remind and motivate you to move more and provide you with feedback on your efforts to do so. Many of the trackers also collect and calculate other useful information, such as heart rate, number of calories burned, and even sleep parameters. Numerous software applications exist for these devices that enhance their usability for health and fitness purposes.

Now, why do we need a gadget to tell us how many steps we take? Because studies have consistently shown that the majority of people can't accurately estimate the amount of physical activity they engage in. Many of us require a monitor, such as a fitness tracker, to provide an objective assessment of how much we actually move or don't move.

So, will a fitness tracker make you healthier? It's debatable. Yes, it gives you objective information. But, just like any monitor, it does nothing to improve your health unless you act on the data it supplies. It's up to you to take advantage of the readings.

You don't need to reach the often-quoted goal of ten thousand steps a day to be healthier. Your goal will depend on a number of factors, including your age, medical conditions, and present state of fitness. Because there are health risks associated with being more active, you should always consult your doctor beforehand about what considerations and limitations exist on increasing the number of steps you take each day.

THINGS TO KNOW FOR HEALTH AND LONGEVITY

62. Physiological monitoring techniques and devices can help you live a healthier and longer life.
63. Your longevity depends on oxygen.
64. Palpating a pulse can save a life or prevent a stroke.
65. Learn to recognize an irregular pulse that may be AFib.
66. Be aware that AFib can present with minimal symptoms.
67. Hypertension, the silent killer, can be unmasked with home blood pressure monitoring.
68. Understand how high blood pressure can damage your body.
69. Apply the pointers on how to measure your blood pressure accurately.
70. Use a pulse oximeter to alert you to low blood oxygen levels.
71. Understand what blood oxygen saturation really is.
72. Apply the pointers on how to use a pulse oximeter.
73. A normal body temperature doesn't completely rule out an infectious process.
74. Use a fitness monitor to provide an objective measurement of your activity level.
75. Monitors provide data that are useless unless understood and acted upon.
76. All monitors have limitations—know and respect them.

NOTE

The techniques and devices in this chapter are not to be used to self-diagnose, treat, or cure any disease or health conditions. They are not intended for any of these purposes.

Monitoring's greatest value lies in its ability to tell you that something is wrong and that you should seek medical care—at times, emergently. Monitoring's greatest danger is that you might not seek medical help because of a normal value. You must recognize that your pulse can be regular, your blood pressure normal, and your oxygen saturation 100 percent even in the face of an active heart attack, stroke, or other life-threatening emergency. If you are experiencing symptoms and are thinking of calling 911, going to the emergency room, or contacting your doctor—then do it. Do not let any monitor readings or interpretations of readings delay or stop you from doing so.

CHAPTER 7

OPERATING ROOM POINTERS FOR BETTER HEALTH

Almost half a year into Eddie's illness, I needed to start an intravenous (IV) line on him. He had become dehydrated and needed IV fluids. The problem was that it was flu season and I had just recently developed cold symptoms. If I had a respiratory infection, the last thing I wanted to do was to spread it to my dad.

To minimize the risk of infecting him, I wore a surgical mask, washed my hands thoroughly with soap and water, and put on a pair of gloves before I entered his living quarters. I then quickly inserted the IV and promptly exited the room.

FROM THE OPERATING ROOM TO HOME USE

The techniques and equipment utilized in operating rooms are designed to protect patients and medical personnel. Some of these same methods and items can also be used at home, in your everyday life, to keep you safe and in good health. They certainly helped Eddie reach his centenarian years.

They may appear simple at times, but a deeper understanding of these measures will aid you in effectively implementing them in the correct situations. With that in mind, let's examine how these techniques and equipment can be applied to living a healthier and longer life.

SLED TO PROTECT AGAINST HARMFUL AGENTS

X-rays are used in surgical suites for a variety of reasons, from visualizing bone fractures, to outlining the kidney's urinary system, to guiding the positioning of wires and catheters in blood vessels. To protect the OR staff from the harmful effects of the X-rays' radiation, we practice something I call **SLED** or Shield, Limit Exposure, and Distance.

S—We shield ourselves from the radiation by wearing lead aprons and lead neck collars.

LE—We limit exposure to the radiation by minimizing X-ray imaging times and the number of X-ray pictures taken.

D—We distance ourselves from the X-ray source to exponentially decrease the amount of radiation reaching us.

When Eddie was bedridden, I was especially concerned about him catching a respiratory infection. In his condition and at his age, he was at a high risk of severe complications and even death. To protect him, the family practiced **SLED**.

At the entrance to his bedroom was a table, where we placed a box of surgical face masks and gloves. Anyone who came by to see him and had symptoms of a cold or flu—sniffles, runny nose, or cough—was requested to wear a mask and don a pair of gloves before entering his living space. The mask and gloves served as shields to minimize the spread of any germs into the room. The visit was kept short to limit exposure time, and visitors stood across the room to distance themselves from my father during their interaction. This practice of **SLED** worked well to protect him from respiratory infections during his recovery—so well that we continued it for the rest of his life.

In the time of COVID-19, the principles of **SLED** have been essential to prevent the spread of the disease. Face masks are worn as a shield to block the dissemination of the virus into the environment. Limited exposure is practiced by quarantining—people only going outside when absolutely necessary. And social distancing is imposed, keeping us apart at a distance of at least six feet, the approximate range most particles can travel as a result of coughing or sneezing. These actions, along with handwashing and the avoidance of touching your mouth, nose, or eyes, all reduce the chance of the virus spreading to you and to others.

But **SLED** is not relevant only during an illness or a pandemic; it can be applied to protect your health in your day-to-day life. The concept has practical applications for staying safe in a variety of situations that threaten your well-being. Let's look at a couple of examples of the application of **SLED**.

A diesel-burning truck spewing dark clouds of potentially carcinogenic exhaust fumes stops next to you. If you are in a car, you can close your windows and press the air recirculation button to shield yourself from the pollutant. But what if you are standing on the sidewalk waiting for a bus that you must catch? Shielding and limiting exposure time may not be possible options, but the use of distance can significantly reduce the amount of fumes you are breathing in. Taking a few steps back to double or triple your distance from the truck may protect you by greatly decreasing the concentration of the pollution you are exposed to.

Suppose you are looking to enjoy an outdoor vacation in a sunny destination but want to minimize the harmful effects of the sun's ultraviolet radiation (UV rays). You are probably applying **SLED**. You put on sunscreen lotion and wear appropriate clothing to shield your skin. You limit exposure time by reducing your hours in the sun, especially during the middle of the day, when the sun is the most intense. You may also use distance to your advantage by avoiding vacation spots closer to the equator. At these locations, the sunlight has a shorter atmospheric distance to travel through, which results in more UV radiation reaching your skin. (You may also want to avoid high altitudes, such as high up in the mountains, where a thinner atmosphere provides less shielding from the UV rays.)

You can apply the concept of **SLED**—Shield, Limit Exposure, and Distance—to reduce your exposure to a variety of harmful agents.

TAKE ADVANTAGE OF THE POWER OF DILUTION

There is a saying that "the solution to pollution is dilution." Surgeons apply this thinking when they clean out pockets of infection from the body. They irrigate the infectious matter in the abdomen, joint, or other body space over and over again with water or saline. Copious amounts of fluid are used to dilute and wash out the infected material.

I used this concept during the time Eddie was unable to move, when he developed small pressure ulcers on his skin despite the family's best efforts to prevent them. If these sites appeared infected, I would repeatedly wash out the areas with sterile saline, diluting and removing the bacteria and debris. This cleaned the bedsores effectively and allowed for better healing.

Let's look at why dilution works so effectively. The power of dilution is evident when we apply a bit of math. Say you have a glass of water with one hundred particles of what we will call "*x*" dissolved completely in it. You spill out 90 percent of the water and refill the glass. The water in the glass now holds ten particles of *x*. You repeat the process, spilling out 90 percent again and then refilling. Now only one particle of *x* remains. By keeping 10 percent of the water and with two cycles of dilution, the amount of *x* is decreased from one hundred to one—or the concentration of *x* is reduced by 99 percent. You can see how dilution is a potent technique to quickly drop the amount and concentration of an unwanted agent.

Other Uses for the Power of Dilution

Treating infected areas and cleaning out wounds are not the only situations in which dilution comes in handy. The power of dilution is what protects you when you distance yourself from sources of air pollution. Consider a cloud of toxic smoke. Doubling your distance from the source may decrease the number of smoke particles that you inhale not by a factor of two, but possibly by a factor of four (2×2), and tripling the distance, by possibly a factor of nine (3×3). That's because as the distance increases, the smoke is diluted into a much larger volume of air. The power of dilution is that it frequently brings about exponential changes.

You may also use the power of dilution for good oral hygiene, which is associated with better overall health. After eating your meals, there are residual sugars and food particles remaining in your mouth that contribute to the formation of plaque. Millions of bacteria in your mouth feed off this substance, causing dental cavities and gum disease. You can help prevent these conditions by removing some of the remaining sugar and food pieces by swishing and rinsing your mouth with water two or three times after eating. This simple action has been shown to protect your enamel, reduce the number of cavities, and improve oral health.

Understanding and taking advantage of the power of dilution can help you stay healthy.

HANDWASHING SAVES LIVES

Germs are the reason we wash our hands. Before the mid-1800s, most doctors believed that diseases were caused by miasma (bad air). They thought that illnesses such as cholera and the plague were brought about by breathing in noxious vapors, such as the air from sewage and rotting matter. It wasn't until the discovery of the germ theory by Louis Pasteur in the early 1860s that doctors began to understand that many diseases were actually brought about by microscopic organisms they called "germs." This was a vital medical revelation that would eventually lead to antibiotics, antiseptic surgical techniques, and vaccines.

In the hospital, healthcare workers are taught the importance of handwashing. They wash their hands before and after patient contact, before and after the use of gloves, and before and after performing procedures. It's one of the most important things they can do to prevent the spread of infectious diseases in a medical setting. At home, it can also play an essential role in keeping you safe from germs.

Germs can't spread by themselves. They must be transmitted from person to person or object to person, and one of the most common vehicles for transmission are the hands. This is true in the hospital and at home. You touch something that has germs and then you touch your nose, mouth, or eyes—vulnerable sites of the body where these microbes can enter. Germs can also be the link to food-borne illnesses when someone prepares food using germ-laden hands.

Singing "Happy Birthday" Twice

Knowing that you must wash your hands frequently is important, but you should also know *how* to wash your hands. Here's the way medical personnel are instructed to do it. Wet your hands with water, apply soap, and lather up. Rub your hands together, making sure you cover your fingers, fingernails, and the back of your hands. To do it correctly, wash for at least twenty seconds before rinsing and drying with a clean towel or cloth. It is commonly taught that singing the "Happy Birthday" song twice covers the necessary time for proper handwashing.

Is Handwashing or Using a Hand Sanitizer More Effective?

Alcohol-based sanitizers do kill many germs and thus play an important role in preventing the spread of infection. They are convenient and can be used when soap and water are not available. That said, sanitizers may not kill some pathogens, such as the norovirus, the common cause of acute gastroenteritis outbreaks in schools and on cruise ships. Moreover, sanitizers are not as effective as washing your hands when your hands are visibly dirty.

Do as we do in the hospital—know when and how to wash your hands and use alcohol-based sanitizers when appropriate. If you're unsure, soap and water is a safer choice than sanitizers.

TWO DIFFERENT FACE MASKS AND THEIR RESPECTIVE USES

The use of surgical face masks began in the early 1900s. Initially, they were made of cotton gauze and worn solely to protect the surgeons. The masks prevented the doctor's nose and face from being splattered or exposed to infectious bodily fluids. Today, people working in operating rooms put on the mask primarily to shield patients from their respiratory and oral secretions—the mask catches bacteria and viruses expelled from the wearer's nose and mouth when they speak, sneeze, or cough.

Because of its loose fit, the surgical mask is not specifically designed to protect you totally from breathing in germs. However, it can still reduce the bacteria and virus load you are exposed to. This is important because the number of germs entering your body may determine whether or not you contract an illness or, if you were to get sick, the severity of the illness. An additional benefit is that the mask may remind you to not touch your mouth or nose. In these ways, a surgical mask provides some degree of protection from respiratory pathogens.

N95 face masks—or N95 respirators, as they are sometimes called—are masks that can filter out 95 percent or more of airborne particles. They have become well known to the public since COVID-19 due to their greater efficiency at shielding healthcare workers from breathing in the virus. Prior to the pandemic, they were utilized infrequently in hospitals and reserved only for use with contagious diseases that are aerosolized, such as tuberculosis, chicken pox, and measles.

To be effective, N95s require a snug facial fit, essentially forming a complete seal around the mouth and nose. If fitted properly and worn correctly, they do offer significant protection against germs and other airborne agents, such as dust, smoke, and other particulate matter—thus their other role as particulate filtering equipment for industrial applications.

While the N95s can shield you from most particulate air pollution, surgical face masks cannot effectively do so. You should avoid exposure to environmental pollutants with them, as studies have shown they offer only a small degree of protection. The material they are composed of and their loose fit make surgical face masks inadequate for this purpose.

DISPOSABLE GLOVES ARE BARRIERS TO GERMS

While I am providing anesthesia in the operating room, my hands can come into contact with blood, oral and nasal secretions, and even cerebral spinal fluid (when I administer a spinal anesthetic). Disposable surgical gloves provide a physical barrier between my hands and these bodily fluids. They are a vital part of my personal protective equipment (PPE).

At home, I use disposable gloves to reduce my exposure to dirt and germs. I put on a pair for numerous purposes—when handling raw meats, taking out the garbage, or cleaning up after my dog. It's a simple and effective way to stop the spread of germs.

To take full advantage of gloves, you must decide on the material and fit, and if they should be powdered or non-powdered. You also need to know how to remove them without contaminating your hands.

How to Select the Material

Disposable gloves can be made from polyethylene, latex, vinyl, or nitrile.

Polyethylene

Polyethylene, or poly, gloves are good for light chores such as food handling. The fit is looser, so these gloves may not be suitable for precise activities such as manipulating small pieces. They are the cheapest of the disposable gloves, and these are the gloves I use when I wipe my dog's paws after a run in the backyard or his backside after he does his business.

Latex

Latex is a natural substance made from rubber. It can provide a comfortable fit, with the retention of good tactile sensation. The major disadvantage of latex is its potential for allergic reactions, including life-threatening anaphylaxis. If you repeatedly wear these gloves, you can increase your risk of developing a latex sensitivity. For this reason, I minimize the use of latex gloves at home.

Vinyl

Vinyl gloves work well in the kitchen and for personal home care activities. They have a better fit and better touch sensitivity than poly gloves, and allergic reactions to this material are rare. They are my first choice for an all-around glove. I use them to take out the garbage and to help in the kitchen.

Nitrile

Nitrile is a synthetic material that allows for superior sensitivity and dexterity. For many wearers, it provides a tight fit, yet it is the most comfortable. It is less allergenic than latex, but there is still allergic potential.

In the operating room, it was my go-to glove when I performed procedures. At home, I use it when I want to be meticulous with my work—for example, gluing together tiny items or, when my father was ill, starting an intravenous line. Its downside is its cost—it is usually the most expensive of the material choices.

Get the Right Fit

In a medical setting, where precise tactile sensation and the movement of the fingers are essential, the fit of the glove is crucial. This is why more than a half dozen surgical glove sizes are available to medical professionals. For general public use, most disposable gloves come in only three sizes: small, medium, and large. You should make sure to choose a size that allows for adequate dexterity to perform your specific tasks safely and effectively.

Powdered or Non-powdered?

Disposable gloves are available powdered or non-powdered. The powdered ones are easier to put on and may reduce sweating in the gloves. These are their main benefits. But for medical use, the FDA banned powdered gloves in 2017 because they posed risks of allergic and inflammatory reactions in patients and healthcare workers. It is recommended that these gloves be avoided if used for health, personal, or food handling purposes. For my home use, I've always preferred the non-powdered variety.

Correct Glove Removal Technique

The correct technique for glove removal (doffing) requires that you don't contaminate your hands with the dirt and pathogens that reside on the outside of the gloves. This is how we do it in the operating room.

Taking off the first glove of the pair is easy. Grasp at or above the wrist and pull down toward your fingers to peel the glove, inside out, off your hand. Removing the second glove is a bit trickier, since the hand doing the doffing is now ungloved and unprotected. The key is to avoid touching any part of the second glove that may be contaminated.

Slip a couple of fingers under the open end of the remaining glove, touching only the glove's inside, which is clean. Using these fingers as a hook, pull downward, toward the fingers, to peel the remaining glove, inside out, off the hand. Be careful not to touch the soiled surface of that glove.

Wash Your Hands Before and After

It is important to know that your disposable gloves may have small defects in them that are not visible to the naked eye. For this reason, it is recommended that you wash your hands before putting on gloves if you intend to handle food or provide personal care. Because of these imperfections and the possibility that hand contamination may occur during glove removal, you should also always wash your hands after taking the gloves off.

Disposable gloves are a handy aid that keeps your hands clean and helps to prevent the transmission of germs.

THINGS TO KNOW FOR HEALTH AND LONGEVITY

77. Apply **SLED** to protect yourself from harmful agents.
78. There is exponential power in repeated dilution.
79. Dilution techniques can reduce your exposure to unhealthy substances.
80. Handwashing is an effective means to stop the transmission of germs.
81. Hand-wash for at least twenty seconds; to count your time, sing the "Happy Birthday" song twice.
82. Recognize when you can effectively use hand sanitizers.
83. Wear a surgical face mask to stop the spread of germs.
84. A surgical face mask only partially protects you from breathing in germs and particulate matter.
85. Wear an N95 mask for greater protection against respiratory agents.
86. An N95 mask must be worn with a snug facial fit to be effective.
87. Use disposable gloves to help prevent the spread of germs.
88. Select the correct glove for your needs, including the appropriate material and fit.
89. Know how to remove the gloves so that you don't contaminate yourself.

CHAPTER 8

STAYING HEALTHY THROUGH YOUR SENIOR YEARS

It was a cool, crisp, fall evening. At 101, my father walked around the backyard with me by his side. His steps were slow and small, and he paused every now and then to look carefully around.

"How are you feeling?" I asked.

"Wonderful." He smiled and pointed to a tree dressed in its bright autumn colors.

"Look at the leaves!" he exclaimed. "They are so beautiful as they grow old, before they die and fall off the trees."

Eddie understood that aging was a part of life. "If you live long, you must grow old," he would say to me in his later years. He embraced his fate and so did not fear it. Instead, it was a happy time for him. For those around my father, it was a beautiful thing to see.

In this final chapter, we'll discuss specific problems that seniors face. Eddie's approach to aging extended his longevity, but more importantly made the later years of his life some of the best. Your twilight years can be wonderful—if you have the right perspective.

DECREASED PHYSIOLOGICAL RESERVES WITH AGING

Soon after Eddie became a centenarian, he was diagnosed with congestive heart failure. His heart was no longer adequately pumping oxygen-filled blood to the tissues in his body. He now felt weaker and fatigued more readily.

"This old car is breaking down," Eddie said to me when he learned of his heart condition. "It's slowing down and needs more repairs."

As you age, there are changes to your major organ systems that decrease your physiological reserves. Eddie was fortunate that, with a healthy lifestyle, good medical care, and some favorable genes, he was able to minimize and delay the decline.

Here are some of the changes typically associated with aging and their health implications:

CARDIOVASCULAR

- Blood pressure increases, and the output of the heart falls as blood vessels stiffen.
- The heart walls thicken, raising the risks of heart failure.
- The cardiac conduction (electrical) system becomes less responsive.

Significance: It's harder to maintain a high level of physical activity. You tire and can become short of breath more quickly. Your heart doesn't respond as readily to exercise or other cardiovascular stressors.

PULMONARY

- The lung tissue loses some of its elasticity, and expiratory flow rates decrease.
- The surface area for oxygen and carbon dioxide gas exchange is reduced.
- Respiratory muscles weaken.
- Pulmonary capacity diminishes.

Significance: It becomes more difficult to move air and oxygenate the body. You don't tolerate the flu, pneumonia, or other acute lung illnesses as well.

NEUROLOGIC

- Brain size shrinks as neurons are lost.
- Neurotransmitter levels drop.
- The speed of neural connections declines.
- Cerebrovascular disease can develop, leading to decreased blood flow to parts of the brain.

Significance: There is a slowing of cognitive processing abilities. The brain becomes more sensitive to pharmaceutical agents. Confusion and disorientation occur more easily.

RENAL

- Blood flow to the kidneys decreases.

- The number of nephrons (filtering units) declines.
- The filtration rate slows.

Significance: The ability to excrete drugs and waste products may be diminished. Problems with water and electrolyte balance occur more frequently.

IMMUNOLOGIC
- Fewer immune cells are produced.
- The immune system is less responsive.
- The ability to detect and destroy cancerous cells diminishes.

Significance: You can develop infections more readily, and their complications can be more severe. Recovery from infections is slower. Your risk of cancer is increased.

Other changes include loss of muscle tissue, thinning of bones, and decreased vision and hearing. The health lesson here is that seniors have less physiological reserves, and because of this, they can't cope with physical stress and sickness as well as those who are younger. If they become acutely ill, expeditious medical treatment is even more important.

MEDICAL CHECKUPS ARE ESSENTIAL

Increased age, by itself, is a major risk factor for many diseases. It makes you more susceptible to the leading causes of death in the United States: heart disease, cancers, respiratory illnesses, and strokes. Because of aging's association with disease, it's crucial for the elderly to keep up with routine medical checkups. You must remember that many illnesses may have few or no symptoms, so wellness doctor visits are still in order to detect these afflictions, even if you look and feel fine.

DON'T ASSUME IT'S BECAUSE OF OLD AGE

Previously, I told you how I assumed it was old age that caused my father to start losing his balance when, in fact, it was from low blood sodium levels. It was a costly mistake to make.

As people grow old, they will develop new symptoms, many of which can appear to be the result of aging—for example, changes in vision, decreased appetite with weight loss, and memory lapses with confusion. Don't assume these and other new, persistent symptoms are just from old age. And don't assume that nothing can be done to treat them.

A senior's deteriorating vision can be the result of cataracts, glaucoma, or macular degeneration, a condition of the retina. Their loss of appetite can be the result of depression, hidden cancers, or something as simple as ill-fitting dentures. And memory lapses and confusion can arise from medication side effects, metabolic disorders, or brain pathology. The causes may be treatable if discovered, and partial or complete resolution of the symptoms may be possible.

THE BODY'S REACTION TO DRUGS CHANGES

When Eddie was approaching his hundredth birthday, I once gave him a small dose of over-the-counter Benadryl to treat some itching from a rash that he had developed. It was only one half of a 25 mg tablet that had been cut into two equal pieces. He took the medication in the morning, and this resulted in him sleeping for most of the day.

Drugs affect the elderly differently. With aging, the brain is more susceptible to pharmaceutical agents. Also, aging extends the half-life of many drugs. Medications tend to hang around longer in the body, continuing to exert their effects. This is because liver and kidney functions are reduced with aging and drugs are not metabolized or excreted as efficiently. Seniors must therefore be careful when taking any medications, especially those with a sedative component—a greater degree of sedation can occur, and this may lead to accidents, such as slips and falls.

Polypharmacy—the use of multiple drugs at the same time—is another pharmacological concern in the elderly. Because of their chronic diseases, seniors frequently are taking a number of prescription drugs; two or three medications may be necessary to manage their hypertension and heart problems, another couple to control diabetes, and a few more to treat elevated cholesterol, arthritis, and osteoporosis. They may even be taking prescribed drugs to treat the side effects of other drugs, such as medications to combat nausea and upset stomach, two common reactions to pharmaceuticals. To further complicate the polypharmacy picture, many people take over-the-counter medicines and supplements.

The problem with taking multiple drugs at the same time is a significant risk of side effects and detrimental interactions between the various medications. Remember that your body is a collection of complex chemical reactions. The more bioactive agents you put into it, the higher the chances of adverse events. Seniors are at a particular risk for confusion and dizziness when they are on multiple medicines. Other serious consequences—abnormalities in blood chemistries, increased bleeding, and changes in blood pressure and heart rate—are also possible.

Here is what you can do to protect yourself from polypharmacy:

- Only take over-the-counter medication and supplements that you need.
- Make a list of all the medications you are on. Include the dosages and how many times a day you take each medicine. Provide the list to your doctors. This is important because you may be seeing multiple medical specialists, and they may be unaware of what medications have been prescribed by others.
- Read the drug information sheet that accompanies each prescription. It can alert you to possible adverse reactions between the medications you are taking. Also, ask your doctors and pharmacists about possible drug interactions.

MANAGING OTHER CONDITIONS ASSOCIATED WITH AGING

Dementia: Take Preventive Steps to Reduce Your Risk

When Eddie was 101 years old, I was sitting next to him when he recalled an event from almost two decades earlier.

"Remember when she stuck her hands into the chocolate cake and started waving them around?" said my father as he laughed, recollecting one of the many antics of his youngest granddaughter.

I had to think hard about it to retrieve the memory. "Oh yeah, I can picture it now. It was her sister's birthday cake."

My dad retained his memory and never developed dementia. People who knew him would tell me that it was because he always kept his mind active and was always learning new things. There may be some truth to this, but it wasn't that simple. Eddie did many other things that contributed to him staying mentally sharp.

To understand why my dad didn't develop dementia, it's important to know what dementia is. It's not a specific disease but, instead, a group of symptoms. Confusion, loss of memory, difficulty with thinking and judgment, and changes in personality and behavior are all parts of this syndrome.

There are many types of dementia, the most common being Alzheimer's. There is an early onset variety that is rare and has a strong genetic link. The more recognized and common version is late onset Alzheimer's, which has only a small genetic component—not everyone with the late onset genes will develop Alzheimer's, and not everyone with the late onset disease will have the Alzheimer's genes.

Vascular dementia is the second most common form of dementia. It's caused by damage to the brain from impaired cerebral blood flow. A history of hypertension, diabetes, stroke, or heart disease increases your risk of this condition.

So, what did Eddie do to keep his cognitive functions intact? Most importantly, he took care of his health by eating right, staying physically active, and not smoking or drinking. What was good for his body was good for his brain. Next, he continued to be mentally active. He remained curious and loved to learn. He would read for hours every day and explored his creative side by drawing and painting. Finally, he kept his mind relaxed by managing stress well and living a life that was as trouble-free as possible. Eddie always said, "A mind can stay healthy only if it has little worries."

Sarcopenia: Prevent Muscle Loss by Staying Physically Active

Sarcopenia is the loss of muscle mass. It commonly occurs as you age and may affect your quality of life, making it difficult for you to perform everyday tasks. It can make you frail and less mobile, and can increase your chances of falling and sustaining fractures. Associated with increased morbidity and mortality, sarcopenia is one of the most common causes of loss of independence in older adults.

There are many reasons why you may develop sarcopenia. Inactivity, insufficient protein intake, and hormonal changes all contribute to the disorder. If you are sedentary, you will typically lose 3 to 5 percent of your muscle tissue per decade after the age of thirty. This loss of muscle accelerates as you enter your seventh and eighth decades of life. In the United States, almost half of the population in their eighties has sarcopenia.

Eddie never had a problem with this condition until his hyponatremic event. Before that, he kept his muscle mass intact by laboring at work, which included operating the clothes pressing machine, into his mid-seventies. After he retired, he remained active by doing housework and gardening. Additionally, thanks to his routine of constantly standing, walking, and climbing stairs, he regularly used and maintained the largest muscle groups in his body, those in the legs and core.

Eddie did develop severe sarcopenia when he was bedridden for a year. He lost a tremendous amount of muscle tissue due to being unable to move or eat enough. His sarcopenia stabilized and improved a half year into his recovery when his appetite improved and he was able to consume more calories. Later, after he regained the use of his muscles and the ability to ambulate, he put back on most of the lost muscle mass.

For you, preventing loss of muscle tissue as you age will require staying physically active and including some form of resistance movements in your activities or exercises. Like Eddie, you don't need to lift weights, although a weight training program may be useful in the fight against this condition. Also, since muscle is constantly being broken down, adequate protein intake is important. The elderly must make sure they are consuming enough of this macronutrient and enough calories in their meals to build back their muscles.

Falling: Measures to Minimize the Risk

Falls are serious, especially for the older population. Falls are the number one cause of fatal and nonfatal injuries for seniors in this country. According to the Centers for Disease Control and Prevention (CDC), it is estimated that one in four Americans aged sixty-five and older will fall each year.

In my anesthesia practice, I have treated many seniors who fell and required emergency surgery. Frequently, they came to the operating room because of a hip fracture, a potentially life-altering injury. Within a year of fracturing a hip, a senior's probability of death more than doubles and permanent lifestyle changes and loss of independence can occur.

Eddie had only one serious fall in his lifetime, and that was off a ladder when he was in his fifties. After he moved into my home, the family didn't want to take any chances that he might fall, so we took important steps to minimize this risk.

Here are the measures we implemented to prevent falling at home:

- provided good lighting, especially leading to the bathroom, where Eddie may need to walk to at night
- placed handrails in and around his shower
- avoided storing his frequently used items on high shelves
- cleaned up loose objects on the floor that could trip him
- made sure the soles of his slippers and shoes were not slippery
- checked that his medications didn't make him dizzy or cause excessive sedation
- stopped him from engaging in activities with a high-risk of falling, such as going outside when there was snow and ice on the ground

REASONS TO LIVE KEEP US ALIVE

For several months after his stroke-like event, Eddie was unable to move. Over time, however, his ability to move gradually came back—initially in his extremities, when he began wiggling his fingers and toes, and then eventually in his arms and legs. After half a year, he started to regain some core strength and was able to assist the family when we had to reposition him on the bed. Soon after this, he was able to sit up completely, and nearly a year after the onset of the illness, he wanted to stand and walk.

To condition and train him to accomplish this feat, I placed a harness around his torso and fastened a rope to it from the pulley system that had been anchored into his bedroom ceiling. I remember his first attempt at standing. I pulled on the rope to support him as he struggled to maintain an upright posture, but his body wouldn't cooperate. His legs buckled as his torso swayed uncontrollably from lack of muscle strength and coordination. The second and third tries were no different. All of this could have discouraged my father, but it didn't. He never gave up, and he continued to give his best effort every time we practiced this maneuver. Little by little, after a couple of months, he miraculously was able to stand on his own and, soon afterward, walk on his own.

Throughout his recovery, my dad was driven by his will to live and, if he lived, his desire to take care of himself again— to be able to feed, walk, and wash himself. He had always been fiercely independent, and he wanted to regain as much autonomy as possible. Without Eddie's motivation to live and get better, I'm sure that he wouldn't have been able to recover so well. In fact, I believe he wouldn't have even survived beyond the first few weeks of his illness.

What pushed Eddie, at ninety-three years of age, to keep on living was that he still had reasons for staying alive. He had his family that he loved, and hobbies and pursuits that he continued to look forward to. This motivated him to not give up on life and to fight on.

Having reasons to live is important as you age. It gives you the will to live and motivates you to stay mentally engaged and physically active. Numerous geriatric studies show that having reasons to keep living is associated with better health, fewer disabilities, and increased longevity.

MAKE YOUR HEALTHCARE WISHES KNOWN

After Eddie's 101st birthday, I once again talked with him about his healthcare wishes. During that past year, his health had deteriorated greatly. With his congestive heart failure progressing and his body weakening, he started to lose his independence again. He now needed assistance to walk and to wash up.

At this stage of his life, Eddie chose not to have any further medical treatment—including any resuscitative efforts. He told me he had had a good long life and understood that death was an inevitable part of living. He accepted it, just as he accepted getting old.

"I am not afraid of dying," he said. "You live and so you must die. You cannot have one without the other."

It is important to have your healthcare wishes known while you are of sound mind. A living will defines what medical treatments and life-sustaining options are acceptable if you are terminally ill or in need of cardiopulmonary resuscitation. It's a legal document with instructions for your preferences for end-of-life medical care when you are no longer able to make these decisions.

A living will may address the following treatment issues:
- mechanical ventilation (support of breathing with a machine)
- placement of a feeding tube
- blood transfusions
- dialysis
- palliative care (including the wish to die at

home, supplementary oxygen, sedative and pain
medications)
- resuscitative care (placement of breathing tube,
chest compressions, electric shocks to the heart)
- body, organ, and tissue donations

On the ninth of May, 2018, Eddie passed away peacefully at home, in his bed. Following his wishes, there was no medical staff attending to him—it was just his family who loved him by his side. We sat next to my dad, held his hands, and talked softly to him as he took his last breaths.

THINGS TO KNOW FOR HEALTH AND LONGEVITY

90. As you age, your body has less physiological reserves.
91. Expeditious medical care is especially important when the elderly become acutely ill.
92. Because age is a major risk factor for many diseases, it is essential that you keep up with your medical checkups, even if you feel fine.
93. Don't assume new symptoms are just a result of aging.
94. Include resistance movements in your activities and eat enough protein to prevent sarcopenia.
95. To decrease your risk of dementia, practice a healthy lifestyle, stay mentally active, and live life with little worries.
96. Be aware of increased sensitivity to sedative drugs.
97. Polypharmacy raises your risks of adverse drug reactions.
98. Provide your doctors with a list of all the drugs, over-the-counter medications, and health supplements that you are taking.
99. Fall-proof your life.
100. Have reasons to live to keep living.

MAKE A COMMITMENT TO YOUR HEALTH

The 101st and final thing to know is very personal to me. Near the end of editing this book for publishing, my family received a devastating piece of news. Our youngest daughter was diagnosed with breast cancer at the age of twenty-four. We were shocked, in disbelief, and deeply saddened—feeling what many other families and loved ones feel when they, too, hear this diagnosis.

The only blessing was that my daughter discovered her cancer early. She was too young for screening mammograms but nevertheless detected the tumor by self-examination. Thankfully, she learned to be aware of her health at this young age. If she hadn't taken the initiative to care for her own well-being, this malignancy could have been discovered much later, changing the prognosis.

The simple act of a breast self-examination can make a great difference in one's health and longevity—so can other cancer screening exams, routine medical checkups, and, of course, a healthy lifestyle. Despite the possibility that any one of us can develop cancer or other serious illnesses, we still do have control over much of our health—in fact, more than ever before.

Don't take your health for granted; make a conscious choice to live your healthiest possible life. Commit to it. Better yet, be like my daughter: make it a mission, a quest, a passion, so that you will remain vigilant and always do what is necessary to attain and stay in good health. And just as with Eddie, you won't have to try to live long. Longevity will naturally follow your healthy ways.

101. Make a conscious choice to live a healthier life—you definitely can improve your health and live longer.